RADIATION PROTECTION FOR RADIOLOGIC TECHNOLOGISTS

Robert Frankel

Certified Health Physicist
Regional Radiological Health Representative
Food and Drug Administration

McGRAW-HILL BOOK COMPANY
A Blakiston Publication

New York St. Louis San Francisco Auckland Düsseldorf Johannesburg
Kuala Lumpur London Mexico Montreal New Delhi Panama
Paris São Paulo Singapore Sydney Tokyo Toronto

NOTICE

Medicine is an ever-changing science. As new research and clinical experience broaden our knowledge, changes in treatment and drug therapy are required. The editors and the publisher of this work have made every effort to ensure that the drug dosage schedules herein are accurate and in accord with the standards accepted at the time of publication. Readers are advised, however, to check the product information sheet included in the package of each drug they plan to administer to be certain that changes have not been made in the recommended dose or in the contraindications for administration. This recommendation is of particular importance in regard to new or infrequently used drugs.

This book was written by Robert Frankel in his private capacity. No official support or endorsement by the Food and Drug Administration or the United States Department of Health, Education, and Welfare is intended or should be inferred.

**Radiation Protection for
Radiologic Technologists**

Copyright © 1976 by McGraw-Hill, Inc. All rights reserved. Printed in the United States of America. No part of this publication may be reproduced, stored in a retrieval system, or transmitted, in any form or by any means, electronic, mechanical, photocopying, recording, or otherwise, without the prior written permission of the publisher.

1 2 3 4 5 6 7 8 9 0   DODO   7 8 3 2 1 0 9 8 7 6

This book was set in Times Roman by Rocappi, Inc. The editors were J. Dereck Jeffers and J. W. Maisel; the cover was designed by Joseph Gillians; the production supervisor was Leroy A. Young. The drawings were done by Svend A. Andersen.
R. R. Donnelley & Sons Company was printer and binder.

Library of Congress Cataloging in Publication Data

Frankel, Robert.
  Radiation protection for radiologic technologists.

  "A Blakiston publication."
  Includes index.
    1. Radiation—Safety measures. 2. Radiation—Physiological effect. 3. Radiography, Medical—Safety measures. I. Title. [DNLM: 1. Radiation protection. WN650 F83r] RA1231.R2F67   616.07'572'028   76-11743
ISBN 0-07-021875-7

To my wife
Sandy
and our sons
Gary and Jay

Contents

Preface

A request that I have frequently received from radiologic technologists following my lectures on radiation protection has been for a copy of my presentation. I have also been asked for a reference which integrates the necessary basics of radiation physics, radiation biology, and radiation protection. Because my lectures have been presented from outline form and I have not been able to identify a single satisfactory reference text on radiation protection, I have not been able to comply with either request.

Many individuals have therefore suggested that I prepare a textbook on radiation protection with special emphasis on diagnostic radiology in order to provide all interested individuals, students, and radiologic technologists and practitioners with the basic knowledge required to minimize excessive radiation exposure to patients and operators.

The book has been developed primarily for the radiologic technology student who has had the necessary background studies in physics, anatomy, and physiology; and it is a complementary, although thorough, textbook in radiation protection. The book is also recommended for practicing radiologic technologists either for an in-service training program of continuing education or for their own review. In addition, practitioners of the healing arts and radiology residents can use the textbook as a basic reference for radiation protection in diagnostic radiology.

I would like to take this opportunity to personally acknowledge the help of Ken E. Lutz, R.T., A.S., and Dorothy L. Smith, R.T., and to thank my many colleagues for their invaluable assistance in the preparation of this book. Their helpful suggestions have been greatly appreciated. The author also wishes to thank the illustrator, Svend A. Andersen, for his clear and concise figures utilized in the book.

Finally, I would like to thank my family for their encouragement, understanding, and patience. Their suggestions and typing and editing of the many drafts to a great extent contributed to the timely completion of this book.

Robert Frankel

Chapter 1

Review of Interaction of X-Rays with Matter; Quantities and Units of Radiation

Objectives

The student reviews the interaction of x-rays with matter and the quantities and units of radiation used in radiation protection applications. The student should

    1 Be acquainted with the basic mechanisms of the various types of interactions

    2 Be able to describe the probability of occurrence of these interactions as a function of photon energy and atomic number of the absorber

    3 Know the quantities and special units of radiation used in radiation protection applications

    4 Understand the interrelationships between the various quantities and units of radiation

INTERACTION OF X-RAYS WITH MATTER

Basic Ionization Processes

For the purposes of this discussion there are three basic ionization processes which can occur when x-rays interact with matter. They are: (1) photoelectric effect, (2) Compton scatter, and (3) pair production.

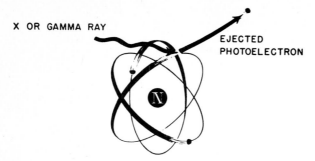

X OR GAMMA RAY

EJECTED
PHOTOELECTRON

Figure 1-1 Photoelectric effect. (Bureau of Radiological Health; Food and Drug Administration; U.S. Department of Health, Education and Welfare.)

Photoelectric Effect In the photoelectric effect, all the energy of the incoming photon is lost and following interaction the photon no longer exists. An analogy to the photoelectric effect is a billiard shot in which the cue ball strikes another ball head on, so that:

a The cue ball suddenly stops, transferring all its kinetic energy to the ball it hit.
b The target ball moves forward in the same direction of travel and with approximately the same velocity (kinetic energy) as had the cue ball.

In the photoelectric effect, the incoming photon interacts with an orbital electron, usually in the innermost orbit (K shell). All the photon's energy is transferred to the orbital electron, so that the photon no longer exists. If the orbital electron acquires sufficient energy, it leaves the influence of the atom and is known as a photoelectron. The atom then has a net charge of plus one, since it has lost a negatively charged electron. The positively charged atom and the negatively charged photoelectron are known as an ion pair. In the above example, the energy of the photon less the energy required to remove the electron from the influence of the atom (binding energy) is equal to the energy of the photoelectron, or

Photoelectron kinetic energy = photon energy − binding energy

Problem If a photon of 38 keV (38,000 eV) interacts with an orbital electron by the photoelectric effect, what will be the initial kinetic energy of the photoelectron if the binding energy of the orbital electron was 4 keV?
Answer

Photoelectron kinetic energy = photon energy − binding energy

Photoelectric kinetic energy $=$ 38 keV $-$ 4 keV

Photoelectric kinetic energy $=$ 34 keV, or 34,000 eV

The rapidly moving photoelectron then interacts with orbital electrons of other atoms. Since like charges repel, some orbital electrons receive sufficient energy in themselves to leave the influence of the atom and form another ion pair. In air, it takes on the average about 34 eV to form one ion pair.

Problem In the above problem, in which the photoelectron had an initial kinetic energy of 34 keV, how many ion pairs will be formed in air?

Answer

$$1 \text{ ion pair} \approx 34 \text{ eV}$$
$$34 \text{ keV, or } 34{,}000 \text{ eV} = \text{? ion pairs}$$
$$\frac{34 \text{ eV}}{1 \text{ ion pair}} = \frac{34{,}000 \text{ eV}}{x \text{ ion pairs}}$$

We then cross-multiply to obtain

$$34x = 34{,}000$$
$$x = 1{,}000 \text{ ion pairs}$$

It is important to note in the above example that from the initial photoelectric ionizing event, a photoelectron was produced that caused an additional 1,000 ionizing events or ion pairs to be formed.

Biological systems depend upon specific molecules which are essential for life. Since the "chemical glue" that holds atoms together to form molecules is electrons, these ionizing events actually can and do break the chemical bonds of the molecules. Therefore, from a single photoelectric interaction with the formation of a high-energy photoelectron, an amplification of hundreds or thousands, or more, can occur. In terms of ion pair production this results in broken chemical bonds with possible adverse biological effects on living systems.

The probability of the photoelectric effect occurring depends on both the energy of the incoming photon and the atomic number (Z number) of the absorber.

Energy There is an inverse relationship between the energy of the incident photon and the probability of photoelectric interaction. In other words, the *greater* the energy of the photon, the *less* the probability of interaction by the photoelectric effect. In tissue (water), the probability of the photoelectric effect is small above energies of 100 keV. However, since in diagnostic radiology most photons are appreciably less than 100 keV, the probability of interaction by the photoelectric effect is the dominant interaction.

Atomic Number (Z Number)   The *greater* the Z number, the *greater* the probability of interaction by the photoelectric effect. The approximate ratio of probability of photoelectric interaction as a function of Z number is about Z^3. This means that if the Z number of a shield is doubled (that is, 2Z), the probability of the photoelectric effect is increased by a factor of Z^3, or $2^3 = 8$ times.

Compton Scatter   In Compton scatter, the incoming photon loses only part of its initial energy to an orbital electron and continues on but in a different direction (scattered). An analogy to Compton scatter is a billiard shot in which the cue ball strikes the target ball off center so that the cue ball goes one way and the target ball goes a different way. The total initial energy of the cue ball is shared between the moving target ball and the "scattered" cue ball.

In Compton scatter, the incoming photon interacts with an orbital electron, usually in an outer orbit. Only part of the photon's energy is transferred to the orbital electron. The photon, which has lost energy in the interaction, continues on although in a new direction. It can then interact with another atom either by the photoelectric effect or again by Compton scatter. In Fig. 1-2 the ejected orbital electron (Compton electron) ionizes other atoms in a manner identical to that of the photoelectron previously discussed.

The sum of the initial energy of the Compton electron plus the binding energy required to remove the orbital electron plus the energy of the scattered photon is equal to the energy of the initial photon. The actual energy

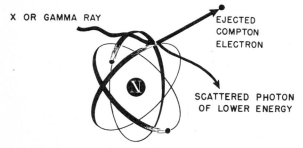

X OR GAMMA RAY

EJECTED
COMPTON
ELECTRON

SCATTERED PHOTON
OF LOWER ENERGY

Figure 1-2   Compton scatter. (Bureau of Radiological Health; Food and Drug Administration; U.S. Department of Health, Education and Welfare.)

of the scattered photon depends on the initial photon energy and the angle through which it is scattered.

As the initial energy of the photons is increased, the scattered photons will be in more of a forward direction. However, at the energies used in diagnostic radiology the photons are primarily backscattered. The minimum scatter in the diagnostic x-ray range occurs at right angles or 90° to the scattering object.

The probability of Compton scatter depends upon the energy of the incoming photon and, to a lesser extent, upon the electron density of the absorber.

Energy The probability of Compton scatter in the diagnostic x-ray range *increases* as the photon energy *increases*. In water, it reaches its peak probability around 500 keV (far above the diagnostic x-ray range) and then decreases.

Electron Density The greater the electron density (electrons per unit mass), the greater the probability of an interaction by Compton scatter.

The electron densities for low *Z* number elements are very similar. However, for the high *Z* number elements electron density decreases. Therefore, the probability of interaction by Compton scatter is approximately the same for light atoms (low *Z* number) but decreases as the *Z* number increases.

Pair Production In pair production, the incoming photon must have an energy greater than 1,020 keV, or 1.02 MeV (far above the diagnostic range). As the photon approaches and interacts with the nucleus of an atom, the energy of the photon is transformed into two particles according to Einstein's reversible formula.

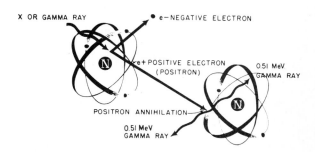

Figure 1-3 Pair production. (Bureau of Radiological Health; Food and Drug Administration; U.S. Department of Health, Education and Welfare.)

$$E \rightleftharpoons mc^2$$

where E = energy
     m = mass
     c = velocity of light

One of the particles formed is a negatively charged electron. The other particle has the same mass but is positively charged. It is known as a positron. If the incoming photon has an energy greater than 1,020 keV, it appears as kinetic energy shared between the electron and the positron. The electron and the positron both interact and ionize other atoms.

Positrons do not exist free in our universe and are known as a form of antimatter; i.e., they will interact and destroy their matter counterparts, electrons, releasing energy in the process.

When a positron collides with an electron, a matter-antimatter annihilation reaction occurs, resulting in the transformation of the mass of both the electron and the positron into energy, two 510-keV (0.51-MeV) gamma photons. The two 510-keV gamma photons will then interact with matter either by the photoelectric effect or by Compton scatter.

The probability of pair production is a function of both the energy of the incident photon and the Z number of the absorber.

Energy   The probability of pair production occurring if the energy of the incoming photon is less than 1,020 keV is absolutely zero. The 1,020 keV energy is the minimum threshold required. However, for practicable applications, energies of 3,000 or more keV are required prior to any appreciable pair production.

Z Number   The *greater* the Z number of the absorber, the *greater* the probability of interaction by pair production.

RADIATION QUANTITIES AND UNITS

The International Commission on Radiation Units and Measurements (ICRU) has established an internationally accepted system of quantities and units suitable for radiation protection applications. The quantities are exposure, absorbed dose, dose equivalent, and activity. The corresponding special units are roentgen, rad, rem, and curie. A quantity is a description of a physical concept, such as distance, while the unit to describe the quantity distance can be the meter.

Exposure (X)

For the purposes of this discussion, the quantity *exposure* can be defined as the absolute value of the total charge of ions of one sign produced in air when the electrons liberated by photons in a volume element of air having a known mass are completely stopped in air.*

The important items to note in discussing the quantity exposure are:

1 It applies only to photons, that is, x-rays or gamma rays.
2 It applies only to their interaction with *air*.
3 The number of electrons formed per unit mass are collected and measured.
4 Therefore, an equation to express the quantity exposure is

$$X = \frac{\Delta Q}{\Delta M}$$

where X = exposure
   ΔQ = coulombs (charge of ions collected)
   ΔM = mass of air, kg

A known mass of air is exposed to photons such that all the ions produced are collected between two charged plates (cathode and anode) and measured. The charge measured is expressed in coulombs. The special unit of the quantity exposure is the roentgen (R). It is defined as

$$1 \text{ R} = 2.58 \times 10^{-4} \text{ coulombs/kilogram}$$

Therefore, if a charge of 2.58×10^{-4} is liberated in 1 kg of air from photons, we say that the *exposure* is 1 R. Please note that a roentgen is defined only in air and applies only to x-ray or gamma-ray photons.

Absorbed Dose (D)

The quantity *absorbed dose* is the mean energy imparted by ionizing radiation per unit mass.†

In the previous definition of exposure we were limited to only photons in air. In absorbed dose, we are speaking of any type of ionizing radiation

---

* For a more precise definition, the reader should read *ICRU Report* 19.
† For a more precise definition, the reader should consult *ICRU Report* 19.

(photons, electrons, neutrons, alpha particles, etc.) as well as their deposition of energy in any media. The special unit for the quantity of absorbed dose is the rad.

1 rad = 100 ergs (unit of energy)/gram (any material)

The material in which the energy is deposited can be living tissue, air, stone, water, etc. Also, the ionizing radiation can be photons, neutrons, alpha particles, etc.

For soft tissue near the surface of the skin, a 1-R exposure in the diagnostic x-ray range will deposit about 87 ergs of energy per gram of tissue, or about 0.87 rad. Therefore, for the purposes of this discussion, we can say that a 1-R exposure approximates an absorbed dose of 1 rad for soft tissue near the surface of the skin.

However, we cannot in this manner approximate the absorbed dose to all tissues of the body. For example, a radiograph may show a clear area under bone, indicating little exposure to the film. Therefore, the bone has absorbed a greater quantity of x-rays (more rads absorbed) than other tissues. This is logical since bone has a much higher effective Z number (because of calcium) than soft tissue. The higher Z number means that x-rays have a much greater probability of interaction in bone by the photoelectric effect (and therefore increased deposition of energy) than in soft tissue.

Dose Equivalent (H)

The quantity *dose equivalent* equates the various types of ionizing radiation in terms of radiation protection applications. The dose equivalent H is equal to the product of the absorbed dose D times a quality factor Q, and times any other modifying factors N.

$$H = DQN$$

where H = dose equivalent
       D = absorbed dose
       Q = quality factor
       N = modifying factor

The quality factor provides the modification due to radiation quality, i.e., deposition of energy per unit length. For example, alpha particles deposit a greater amount of energy per unit length or in a given length of tissue than x-rays. Therefore, the quality factor Q for alpha is greater than for x-rays.

The quality factor for x-rays in the diagnostic range is 1. The modifying factor N is the product of all other modifying factors. At present, it is assigned a value of 1 for all irradiations by external sources.

The special unit for dose equivalent is the rem. Since a quality factor of 1 has been assigned for diagnostic-range x-rays, an absorbed dose of 1 rad will be equal to

$$H = DQN$$
$$H = 1 \text{ rad} \times 1 \times 1$$
$$H = 1 \text{ rem}$$

By expressing dose equivalent in rems, 1 rem of x-rays will equal 1 rem of neutrons, which will equal 1 rem of alpha radiation in terms of radiation protection applications.

Since we have previously stated that an exposure (X) of 1 R of diagnostic-range x-rays will deliver an absorbed dose (D) of approximately 1 rad to soft tissue near the surface of the skin, which is approximately equal to a dose equivalent (H) of 1 rem, the following is numerically true for such soft-tissue exposure:

$$\underset{\text{Exposure}}{1 \text{ roentgen}} \approx \underset{\text{Absorbed dose}}{1 \text{ rad}} \approx \underset{\text{Dose equivalent}}{1 \text{ rem}}$$

Activity (A)

The quantity *activity* is the number of spontaneous nuclear transformations which occur in a radiative material per time interval.

Table 1-1 Summary of Radiation Quantities and Units

Quantity	Symbol	Special unit	Measuring media	Effect measured	Types of applicable radiation
Exposure	X	roentgen (R)	Air	Air ionizations	X or γ only
Absorbed dose	D	rad	Any media	Energy deposited	All ionizing radiation
Dose equivalent	H	rem	Living systems	Biological effects	All ionizing radiation
Activity	A	curie (Ci)	—	Disintegrations per second	All radio-active material

The special unit of activity is the curie (Ci) which is equal to 3.7×10^{10} disintegrations (spontaneous nuclear transformations) per second.

Historically, a curie is approximately equal to the activity of 1 g of ^{226}Ra.

Since a curie (Ci) is a rather large unit, we normally use, in nuclear medicine, the millicurie (mCi), which is one-thousandth of a curie, or the microcurie (μCi), which is one-millionth of a curie.

There is no direct relationship between the quantity activity and the quantities of exposure, absorbed dose, and dose equivalent, which depend not only on activity but also on the type of particles or photons released and their energy.

QUESTIONS

1-1   In the diagnostic x-ray range, what is the predominant type of interaction of x-rays with matter? Will the probability of this effect increase or decrease as the atomic number (Z number) of the absorber is increased?

1-2   What is the threshold energy required for pair production to occur? Is this energy within the diagnostic x-ray range?

1-3   Is it correct to say that the bone received a dose of 1R? Why?

1-4   What is the atomic number (Z number) of barium? Why is barium part of certain contrast media? Could sodium be substituted for barium in a contrast media? Explain your answer.

1-5   Explain what happens to the probability on Compton scatter as a function of photon energy.

1-6   If the quality factor Q for fast neutrons is 10, what would be the dose equivalent (rems) of 5 rads of absorbed dose?

1-7   If the quality factor Q for x-rays is 1, what would be the dose equivalent (rems) of 5 rads of absorbed dose?

1-8   Although x-rays in the diagnostic range scatter at all angles, what is the predominant direction of such scatter? At what angle from the scattering object will there be minimum scatter?

1-9   List the special units for the quantities listed below.
　　　　　Absorbed dose
　　　　　Exposure
　　　　　Activity
　　　　　Dose equivalent

1-10   Explain why lead is a more efficient shield than aluminum.

REFERENCES

1   International Commission on Radiation Units and Measurements (ICRU): Radiation Quantities and Units, *ICRU Report* 19, Washington, D.C., 1971.

2   Oman, R.: "An Introduction to Radiologic Science," McGraw-Hill, New York, 1975.

3   Moe, H. J., et al.: "Radiation Safety Technician Training Course Manual," ANL-7291, Rev. 1, National Information Service, U.S. Department of Commerce, 1972.

4   Cember, H.: "Introduction to Health Physics," Pergamon, New York, 1969.

5   Blatz, H.: "Radiation Hygiene Handbook," McGraw-Hill, New York, 1959.

6   Andrews, H.: "Radiation Biophysics," Prentice-Hall, Englewood Cliffs, N.J., 1962.

7   Kaplan, I.: "Nuclear Physics," Addison-Wesley, Reading, Mass., 1963.

8   "X-Ray Interaction with Matter," U.S. Public Health Service, FDA, BRH, training fascicle TP-335, 1967.

Biological Effects of Ionizing Radiation— Basic Mechanisms and Short-Term Effects

Objectives

The student learns the basic mechanisms and short-term effects of ionizing radiation. The student should

  1 Know the basic components of animal cells as they relate to radiation biology
  2 Be able to distinguish between the direct-hit and indirect-hit theories of radiation effects
  3 Understand the relationship of cell sensitivity to cell specialization and rate of division
  4 Acquire the ability to describe dose-response curves and the concept of $LD_{50/30}$
  5 Be aware of the effect of radiation as a function of dose and area exposed
  6 Be able to describe the mechanisms of radiation-induced death

CELL COMPONENTS

Animal cells consist of a nucleus and cytoplasm. The nucleus contains most of the cell's genetic material. The cytoplasm contains many structures of the cell which are essential to metabolism and protein synthesis. A typical animal cell is illustrated in Fig. 2-1.

Cytoplasm

Of the many structures within the cytoplasm, the *ribosomes* are of particular interest in terms of radiation protection applications.

Ribosomes are essential for the manufacture of proteins from amino acids. The actual synthesis of protein occurs within the ribosome itself.

Nucleus

During certain stages of cell division, chromosomes in a cell nucleus can be seen with a light microscope. During other stages they "disappear," and the nucleus appears to be an irregular granular mass of varying density. Chromosomes contain the genes which are the genetic blueprints for the cells. There are approximately 30,000 genes in a human cell. It is now known that insofar as genetic material is concerned the entire chromosome is composed of genes and, in fact, the genes themselves are composed of a single molecule, deoxyribonucleic acid (DNA). Therefore the chromosome itself is composed of this organic long-chain molecule.

Human cells contain 23 matched pairs of chromosomes. A typical chromosome looks like a small rod. As stated above, this rodlike appearance of the chromosome manifests itself only during specific stages of cell division.

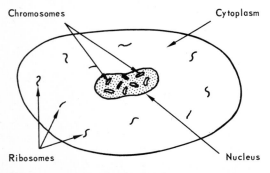

Figure 2-1 Typical animal cell.

By the use of an electron microscope it has been determined that the long-chain molecule of DNA condenses like a spring so that it appears to be a rod. This is illustrated in Fig. 2-2. The length of the DNA molecule is more than 150 times the length of the chromosome.

Further investigation has shown that the DNA molecule itself is not in the form of a single strand but is double-stranded in a manner similar to a rope ladder with cross-connections. In addition, it is coiled around to form a double helix. This is analogous to a rubber band attached to a propeller of a

DNA

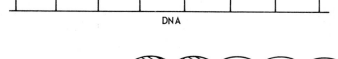

Long DNA Molecule   Coil of tightly condensed DNA
                                which appears as a
                                Rod Shaped Chromosome

Figure 2-2 DNA—forms.

DOUBLE STRAND, DOUBLE HELIX
DNA

DNA

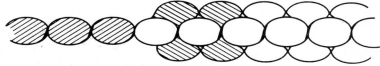

Double Helix DNA in a coil of 20-30 Nanometers

Figure 2-3 DNA—double helix.

model airplane. The two strands of the rubber band represent the double-stranded DNA molecule. As the propeller is wound up, the rubber band coils around itself to form a helix; further winding of the propeller would cause the rubber band to coil around the previous coils, forming a double helix. DNA exists in a cell as a double helix, as shown in Fig. 2-3.

Since the chromosomes are composed of genes, which are DNA molecules, if anything happens to the chromosomes to alter or destroy a specific gene, the function of the cell which was controlled by the gene will be impaired or modified. If the particular function was essential for the normal life of the cell, the cell may either die or continue to exist in an abnormal manner.

CELL RADIATION EXPOSURE

Direct-Hit Theory

If the nucleus of a cell is exposed to ionizing radiation, interactions occur. As illustrated in Fig. 2-4, if the interaction occurs *directly* on the DNA molecule, the resulting ionization can break a chemical bond. This is known as the direct-hit theory. Further exposure can cause additional breaks in the "rope ladder" structure of DNA. There will not be any physical change in the chromosome's appearance from direct hits widely spaced through its length.

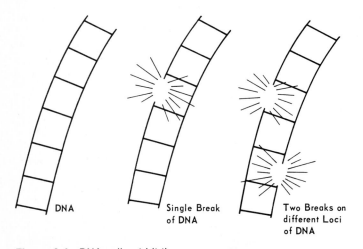

DNA

Single Break
of DNA

Two Breaks on
different Loci
of DNA

Figure 2-4 DNA—direct-hit theory.

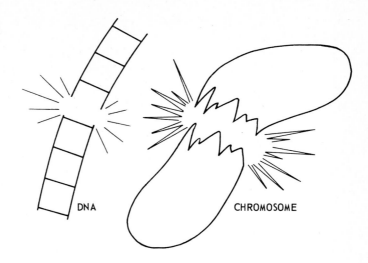

Figure 2-5 DNA—chromosome cleavage.

If, as in Fig. 2-5, two direct hits occur in the same "rung" of the DNA rope ladder, the molecule itself is actually broken in half and the chromosome will appear to be cleaved or broken.

If the abnormally cleaved chromosome divides, each new daughter cell will receive an incorrect amount of genetic material, which can lead to its death or impaired function. Although abnormal chromosome cleavage from direct hits can and does occur, the probability of its occurrence is far too small to explain all the effects of ionizing radiation.

Indirect-Hit Theory

Water Ionization Cells are composed of approximately 85 percent water. When water is exposed to ionizing radiation, ions are formed, H_2O^+ plus an electron.

$$H_2O \rightarrow H_2O^+ + _{-1}^{0}e$$

The H_2O^+ dissociates almost immediately (10^{-11} sec) to form a hydrogen ion plus a *free hydroxy radical*.

$$H_2O^+ \rightarrow OH\cdot + H^+$$

Free	Hydrogen ion
hydroxy	
radical	

A *free radical* is a chemical molecule which has an unpaired electron and is thus highly unstable. It tries to "take" an electron from a different molecule, which oxidizes the other molecule. Therefore, free radicals are oxidizing agents. The free hydroxy radicals can combine to form H_2O_2 (hydrogen peroxide) which in the alkaline media of cells acts as an oxidizing agent.

$$OH\cdot \; + \; OH\cdot \; \rightarrow \; H_2O_2$$

The electron from the initial water interaction ($_{-1}^{0}e$) combines with a water molecule to form H_2O^-.

$$H_2O \; + \; _{-1}^{0}e \; \rightarrow \; H_2O^-$$

The H_2O^- dissociates to form a hydrogen atom plus a hydroxyl ion:

$$H_2O^- \; \rightarrow \; H\cdot \; + \; OH^-$$
$$\text{Hydrogen} \quad \text{Hydroxyl ion}$$
$$\text{atom}$$

The hydrogen atom will combine with oxygen to form a perhydroxyl free radical.

$$H\cdot \; + \; O_2 \; \rightarrow \; HO_2\cdot$$
$$\text{Perhydroxyl free radical}$$

The initial ionization of water can be summarized as:

$$H_2O \; \rightarrow \; OH\cdot \; + \; H_2O_2 \; + \; H\cdot \; + \; HO_2\cdot$$

Note that three of the products formed ($OH\cdot$, H_2O_2, and $HO_2\cdot$) are oxidizing agents.

Free Radical Reactions   In the direct-hit theory, the initial interaction must occur at or near a DNA strand. In the indirect-hit theory, the interaction does not have to occur in such close proximity to the DNA. Instead the free radicals formed may migrate to the DNA (as well as to other structures) and upon interaction chemically oxidize and destroy parts of the DNA molecule, thereby also destroying genes. The effect of this oxidation may become manifest almost immediately if enough DNA (or a critical gene) is destroyed, or may not become apparent until later cell division, when un-equal amounts of DNA from the fragmented chromosomes are found in each daughter cell.

REPAIR

The existence of a repair mechanism for mammals is obvious in that they do recover from symptoms of the acute radiation syndrome. However, as shown in Fig. 2-6, the extent of the recovery is not necessarily complete insofar as some nonrepairable components are concerned. Experiments on mammals indicate that if a certain quantity of radiation is required to cause a specific effect, a lesser quantity of radiation to the same animal is required to again cause the effect, indicating the existence of some irreparable injury.

Note that every injury is rapidly repaired at first, but there is an accu-mulated irreparable component. If, through carelessness or ignorance, re-peated injuries occur, there can be a buildup of accumulated irreparable damage. As a rule of thumb, approximately 90 percent of the injuries caused by ionizing radiation is repaired, leaving a 10 percent residue of accumu-lated irreparable damage.

CELL SENSITIVITY

The cells of the body that make up the organs and organ systems are differ-ent not only in terms of appearance, but also in their rate of division (mitotic

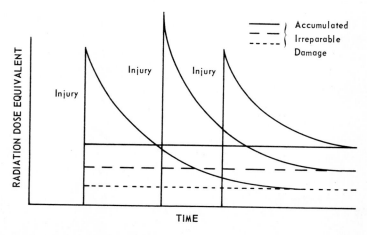

Figure 2-6 Repair concept.

rate) and their metabolism. Early experiments also indicated that not all cells of the body were equally sensitive to ionizing radiation. In 1906, Bergonié and Tribondeau developed their theory concerning cell sensitivity which can be summarized as:

1   "Simple" cells are among the most sensitive cells to ionizing radiation.
2   Rapidly dividing cells are among the most sensitive cells to ionizing radiation.

Among the many complex cells of the body, certain blood cells, particularly blood precursor cells which will eventually become white or red cells, are very "simple" structures. Other cells such as smooth muscle cells, heart cells, liver cells, etc., are more complex. Some of the most complex looking are nerve cells, which have axons and dendrites.

Cells are also multiplying at different rates; e.g., blood precursor cells are rapidly multiplying, becoming more specialized until they finally mature as white or red blood cells (erythrocytes). Other cells have a lower mitotic rate. A nerve cell *after birth* has a mitotic rate of zero. If the cell is destroyed, it is not replaced.

Insofar as acute effects are concerned, the most sensitive cells in the body are the lymphocytes (a type of white blood cell). A whole-body dose of 30 rads will cause a transitory decrease in the lymphocyte count. Other cells in the body are more radioresistant; e.g., 200 rads will prevent the stomach from emptying completely, while a 3,500-rad dose to the liver has no apparent short-term effect.

The most insensitive system is the central nervous system (CNS) after birth. Both the sensitivity of the blood precursor cells and the insensitivity of CNS cells are consistent with the theory of Bergonié and Tribondeau.

The amount of oxygen in the irradiated tissue also directly affects response. As previously discussed, one of the ionization products produced by the irradiation of water is a hydrogen atom. If oxygen is present, $HO_2 \cdot$ is formed.

$$H \cdot + O_2 \rightleftharpoons HO_2 \cdot$$

Cell sensitivity to x-rays increases as oxygen tension is increased. Figure 2-7 shows that the maximum sensitivity is reached at about 20 mm of mercury pressure. It reaches half of its maximum sensitivity at about 2 mm of mercury pressure.

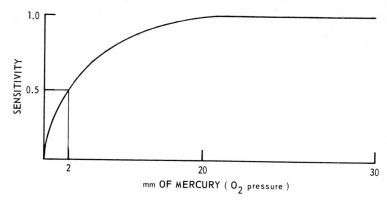

Figure 2-7 Radiation sensitivity—oxygen relationship.

This is why in order to facilitate the effect of radiation, oxygen tension is increased in certain treatment plans for radiotherapy.

DOSE-RESPONSE CURVES

There are currently two major concepts of dose-response curves for ionizing-radiation effects.

Sigmoid Dose-Response Curve

The sigmoid dose-response curve (Fig. 2-8) appears to be of the correct shape for many types of somatic effects, i.e., those which will _not_ be passed on to the individual's children.

As the dose decreases, the response also decreases until there is a dose below which there is no response (threshold). Many types of somatic responses do appear to follow this concept, including death, epilation (loss of hair), and erythema.

If this is the correct concept for all responses, then all that has to be done in terms of radiation protection is to keep the unnecessary radiation dose to less than the threshold level.

However, most experts agree that the sigmoid curve is _not_ the correct shape for the genetic effects of ionizing radiation or for certain types of somatic responses, like leukemia. Instead, the form of the dose-response curve for these responses may be a straight line, as shown in Fig. 2-9.

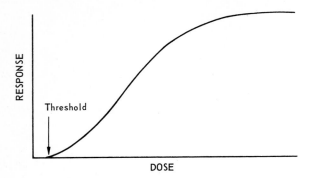

Figure 2-8 Sigmoid dose-response curve.

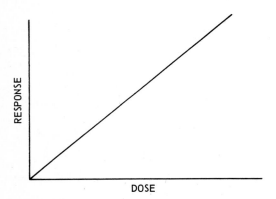

Figure 2-9 Linear dose-response curve.

Linear Dose-Response Curve

In the straight line or linear relationship curve, there is no threshold. This means that if the linear relationship is the correct shape of the dose-response curve, then there is no level of radiation exposure that is absolutely safe. Every exposure involves a risk, albeit an extremely small one if the exposure is also small. In theory, one photon could cause a mutation. However, the probability of such an occurrence is minute compared to the benefit of radiation properly used. Therefore, it is the purpose of this textbook to acquaint the reader with both the necessity and the means of minimizing unnecessary radiation exposure consistent with the best possible use of such radiation. Which of the two curves or combination of them is correct for the low-dose, low-energy x-rays used in diagnostic radiology is still not absolutely certain. In either case, the proper public health approach to this question is to minimize exposure consistent with the best possible results.

WHOLE-BODY RESPONSE

The effect on the whole body depends not only on the dose but also on the dose rate and the area of the body exposed.

Dose Rate If a dose of radiation is fractionated over a period of time, the acute effect on the body will be less than if delivered as a single dose. This is because the body has the opportunity to repair damage due to the fractionated doses.

Area If a large whole-body dose (500 rads) is delivered to a mammal, the prognosis is guarded. However, if the same 500 rads is delivered to a small part of the body (shielding the blood-forming organs), the effect will be minimal.

LD$_{50/30}$ The term LD$_{50/30}$ means lethal dose for 50 percent of the population so exposed within 30 days. The whole-body LD$_{50/30}$ for the adult human population is approximately 450 rems. As illustrated in Fig. 2-10, if

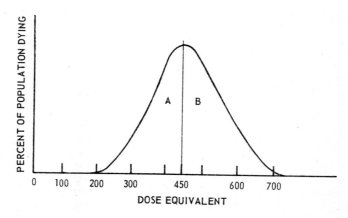

Figure 2-10 LD$_{50}$ concept.

a large number of individuals received a dose equivalent of 450 rems, half of the population so exposed would die within 30 days.

At 450 rems half of the population as represented under part A will die. In addition, some very susceptible individuals will expire at approximately 200 rems.

As the dose equivalent increases past 450 rems, the number of individuals still living after 30 days decreases. At approximately 700 rems, the entire population will have expired within 30 days after exposure.

Acute Radiation Syndrome   The acute radiation syndrome can be divided into four major stages. They are:

1   Initial stage
2   Latent stage
3   Manifest illness stage
4   Recovery or death stage

The following chart summarizes the effects resulting from acute whole-body external exposure of radiation to man.

The dose equivalent of 200 to 300 rems is the minimum required in order for all four stages of the acute radiation syndrome to be seen.

Mechanisms of Mammalian Death   As shown in Fig. 2-11, there appear to be three basic mechanisms of mammalian death from ionizing radi-

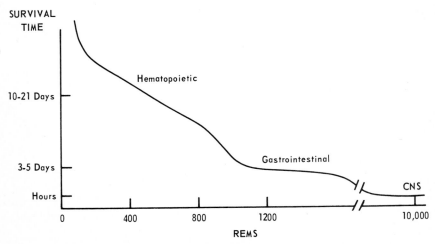

Figure 2-11   Mechanism of mammalian radiation death.

Table 2-1 Summary of Effects Resulting from Acute Whole-Body External Exposure of Radiation to Man

0 to 25 rems	25 to 100 rems	100 to 200 rems	200 to 300 rems	300 to 600 rems	600 rems or more
No detectable clinical effects	Slight transient reductions in lymphocytes and neutrophils	Nausea and fatigue, with possible vomiting above 125 rems	Nausea and vomiting on first day	Nausea, vomiting, and diarrhea in first few hours	Nausea, vomiting, and diarrhea in first few hours
Delayed effects may occur	Disabling sickness not common, exposed individuals should be able to proceed with usual duties	Reduction in lymphocytes and neutrophils with delayed recovery	Latent period up to 2 weeks or perhaps longer	Latent period with no definite symptoms, perhaps as long as 1 week	Short latent period with no definite symptoms in some cases during first week
	Delayed effects possible, but serious effects on average individual very improbable	Delayed effects may shorten life expectancy in the order of 1 percent	Following latent symptoms appear but are not severe: loss of appetite, and general malaise, sore throat, pallor, petechiae, diarrhea, moderate emaciation	Epilation, loss of appetite, general malaise, and fever during second week, followed by hemorrhage, purpura, petechiae, inflammation of mouth and throat, diarrhea, and emaciation in the third week	Diarrhea, hemorrhage, purpura, inflammation of mouth and throat, fever toward end of first week
			Recovery likely in about 3 months unless complicated by poor previous health, superimposed injuries, or infections	Some deaths in 2 to 6 weeks. Possible eventual death to 50 percent of the exposed individuals for about 450 rems	Rapid emaciation and death as early as the second week with possible eventual death of up to 100 percent of exposed individuals

Source: Adapted from "Medical Aspects of Radiation Accidents," U.S. AEC-1963.

ation: hematopoietic (blood) death, gastrointestinal death, central nervous system death.

Hematopoietic Death   At a whole-body dose equivalent of approximately 350 to 1,000 rems, death occurs in about 10 to 21 days. At this dose equivalent, the blood precursors are affected such that they no longer produce new white blood cells. This means that the body has lost the first line of defense against foreign antigens, the process of phagocytosis (the ability of white blood cells to ingest foreign antigens).

The body has also lost the second line of defense against foreign antigens in that the body's large lymphocytes, which produce antibodies, are very sensitive to ionizing radiation and therefore are no longer found in the circulating blood.

The individual is now extremely susceptible to bacterial or viral antigens and has lost or is losing the natural ability to combat infections.

The body has a type of blood cell known as a megakaryocyte. As the cell matures, it fragments to form blood platelets, which in combination with menadione and thrombin are essential for the clotting of blood. Following a large dose of radiation, the production of megakaryocytes is inhibited so that the blood platelet count falls. If the dose is large enough (greater than 300 to 400 rads), subcutaneous bleeding (petechiae) can occur as well as bleeding from the various orifices of the body. Death from a whole-body dose of 350 to 1,000 rems usually occurs following fever, bleeding, etc., in 10 to 21 days.

Gastrointestinal Death   If the dose equivalent to the gastrointestinal tract is approximately 1,000 to 10,000 rems, death can occur in 3 to 5 days.

As illustrated in Fig. 2-12, the lumen of the GI tract is highly convoluted in order to permit the maximum surface area for the absorption of

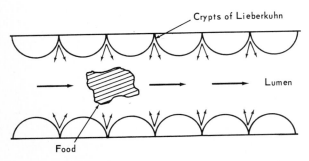

Figure 2-12   GI tract.

food. In Lieberkühn's glands, simple cells, not as simple as blood precursor cells, are rapidly multiplying, pushing out, and becoming more specialized in order to replace those cells which are worn away by the normal passage of food through the GI tract. Following a large radiation dose, the cells in Lieberkühn's glands shut down in mitosis. This means that the GI tract cells which are destroyed are not replaced, resulting in GI ulcers.

Since the body has lost or is losing the ability to clot blood, bleeding occurs into the GI tract. Also, the body is losing proteins, buffers, electrolytes, and other materials directly into the gastrointestinal tract.

Bacteria, yeast, etc., normally found in the GI tract have a direct invasion route through the ulcers, and the body loses the ability to combat these foreign antigens.

A bloody diarrhea occurs with death of the animal in about 3 to 5 days.

Central Nervous System Death The CNS after birth is among the most radioresistant systems in the body to ionizing radiation. But if a dose equivalent of 10,000 rems or more is received, death occurs in just a matter of hours. The cause of death appears to be a malfunction of the neuron sodium pump resulting in motor incoordination, ataxia, hyperexcitability, intermittent stupor, and finally death due to cardiovascular collapse.

DISCUSSION

The situations described in this chapter should never be encountered in the professional career of a diagnostic radiation worker. However, if such a situation does occur and the individual survives, the long-term effects described in the next chapter should be considered. The possibility of long-term effects should also be considered in the case of individuals who receive repeated small exposures to ionizing radiation, no one of which is sufficient to cause any of the short-term effects discussed in this chapter.

QUESTIONS

2-1 Describe the indirect-hit theory as it affects DNA.

2-2 Does a radiation worker acquire an immunity to radiation similar to a typical antigen-antibody immunity? Explain your answer.

2-3 If in a particular animal experiment 300 rads causes epilation, approximate the dose required following complete recovery to cause another epilation to the same animal.

2-4 Why, according to the theory of Bergonié and Tribondeau, are blood precursor cells more sensitive to ionizing radiation than central nervous system cells?

2-5 In certain radiation therapy situations, extra oxygen tension is supplied to the tissue. Why?

2-6 What shaped curve is commonly expected for genetic dose response?

2-7 What response should be taken if a film badge or TLD (thermoluminescent dosimeter) is interpreted as 500 rems?

2-8 What are the four stages of the acute radiation syndrome? Are all four stages apparent at 100 rems?

2-9 What are the three major mechanisms of radiation-induced death?

2-10 Why does bleeding occur in the 300 to 400 rads dose range?

REFERENCES

1   Schultz, R. J.: "Primer of Radiobiology," GAF Publication 6540-009, 1971.

2   Kirk, D.: "Biology Today," Random House, New York, 1975.

3   Bacq, Z. M., and P. Alexander: "Fundamentals of Radiobiology," Pergamon, New York, 1961.

4   Oman, R. M.: "An Introduction to Radiologic Science," McGraw-Hill, New York, 1975.

5   Hollaender, A.: "Radiation Protection and Recovery," Pergamon, New York, 1960.

6   Cember, H.: "Introduction to Health Physics," Pergamon, New York, 1969.

7   "Diagnosis and Treatment of Acute Radiation Injury," International Atomic Energy Agency, International Documents Service, 1961.

8   National Council on Radiation Protection and Measurements: Review of the Current State of Radiation Protection Philosophy, *NCRP Report* 43, 1975.

9   Andrews, H. L.: "Radiation Biophysics," Prentice-Hall, Englewood Cliffs, N.J., 1961.

10 Moe, H. J., et al.: "Radiation Safety Technician Training Course," ANL-7291, Rev. 1, National Information Service, 1972.

11 Saenger, Eugene L., M.D.: "Medical Aspects of Radiation Accidents," U.S. Atomic Energy Commission, 1963.

Chapter 3

Biological Effects of Ionizing Radiation— Long-Term Somatic Effects

Objectives

The student develops an understanding of the possible long-term somatic biological effects from ionizing radiation. The student should

    1 Know four possible long-term somatic effects
    2 Be able to describe several carcinogenic effects due to ionizing radiation
    3 Understand the relationship between the periods of pregnancy and the possible effect of radiation to the developing embryo
    4 Be aware of possible cataractogenic effects
    5 Be conscious of possible life-span shortening effects from ionizing radiation

INTRODUCTION

The previous chapter discussed potential short-term effects from massive acute doses of ionizing radiation. This chapter will describe potential long-term somatic effects. These are the effects which take place in the individual who receives the radiation and cannot be passed on to future generations. They can occur months or many years after recovery from the acute effects of a large dose of radiation, *or* from small doses, no one of which is sufficient to cause any of the short-term effects discussed in the previous chapter. The next chapter will discuss the possible long-term genetic effects of ionizing radiation, i.e., those which can be transmitted to future generations.

It is to be emphasized that even if a mammal were to receive a large dose or many small doses of radiation, the possibility of any of the long-term effects developing is of a statistical nature. That is, just because a radiation dose has been received, this does *not* necessarily mean that the individual will develop any of the possible long-term effects of ionizing radiation. However, in terms of statistics, he has a greater probability of its occurring. An example of this philosophy is cigarette smoking. Just because an individual smokes cigarettes does not necessarily mean that lung cancer will develop, but the individual has a greater probability of developing the disease than the nonsmoking population.

TYPES OF POSSIBLE LONG-TERM SOMATIC EFFECTS

There are four major types of possible somatic effects which have been observed from ionizing radiation. They are carcinogenesis, embryological effect, cataractogenesis, and life-span shortening.

Carcinogenesis

Ionizing radiation in doses greater than 100 rads has been shown to increase the risk of tumors in many species of laboratory animals. What the risk is at lower doses is currently unclear. Using laboratory animals, a linear (straight-line) dose-effect response is seen using high doses and high dose rates of ionizing radiation. If low doses of ionizing radiation are given, the actual shape of the dose-effect curve becomes controversial. It is the contention of some scientists that under the conditions of low dose the carcinogenesis dose-effect curve is either sigmoid or curvilinear. Three types of possible dose-effect curves are shown in Fig. 3-1.

Epidemiological studies and observations of irradiated humans have demonstrated consistently the carcinogenic effects of ionizing radiation. Several of these studies are listed below.

Radium-Dial Painters   During approximately the first 20 years of this century, the East Coast of the United States had a thriving radium-dial-

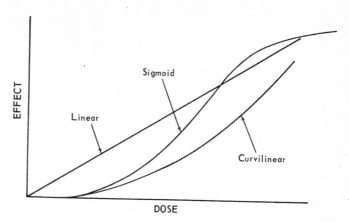

Figure 3-1 Possible dose-effect curves.

painting industry. The factories employed young girls to hand-paint dials with a radium-containing paint, using fine sable brushes.

In order to paint a series of dots (on the dial) which in the dark appeared as a number, some of the girls were taught to "draw" the brush to a fine point using their lips and tongue and then to dip it into the radium paint. The individuals who practiced this technique ingested large quantities of radium. A number of these girls died from the acute effects of radiation. That is, the radium, which is chemically similar to calcium, was concentrated in the bone. The radiation from the radium killed both bone marrow and bone cells, resulting in bone absorption and precipitously low levels of blood cells which led to infections, hemorrhages, and in some cases death.

The U.S. Public Health Service followed the survivors for many years and noted an increased incidence of bone sarcomas as well as other types of cancer from the radium accumulated in the bones.

Thyroid Nodules   Until about 1940, it was an accepted practice to radiograph the thymus gland of an infant with respiratory distress. If the thymus appeared to be enlarged, a therapeutic quantity of x-rays was given in order to shrink the lymphatic tissue of the thymus gland. Since the adjacent organ to the thymus is the thyroid, these patients also received a large quantity of x-rays to their thyroids.

Epidemiological studies by Pifer and Hemplemann, as well as others, have indicated a statistically significant relationship between the development of thyroid cancer and other malignancies of the neck and head areas and the patients' earlier thymus irradiation. The latent period between the original thymus irradiation and the onset of the disease was greater than 10 years.

Studies of patients who were irradiated for other benign conditions of the neck area (tonsillitis, acne, impetigo, etc.) also indicate an association between the irradiation and thyroid tumors. In one such study,[5] the patients developed the tumors an average of 20 years following x-ray exposure.

Medical Radiation Personnel   Some early radiation users, largely due to a lack of knowledge of radiation effects, were exposed to large amounts of radiation. These exposures resulted in an increased number of operator cancer deaths. Skin cancer was one of the major findings among these individuals. In addition, finger lesions were noted in a number of dentists who routinely held film in the patient's mouth.

With increased knowledge of possible risks of radiation, there have been improved radiation protection practices. A more recent study of dentists indicated that their leukemia rate was similar to the rest of the United States population. However, other studies have indicated that there still is a statistically significant increase in the incidence of leukemia to radiologists as compared with physicians who do not use radiation.[7,8]

Children Irradiated In Vivo   Although a more detailed discussion of this topic will be found in the next section of this chapter, it should be stated here that studies have indicated an increased risk of leukemia among young children whose mothers received pelvic x-rays during pregnancy.

Other Human Examples

a   Uranium miners who inhaled radioactive radon gas in the course of their employment had an increased incidence of lung cancer.
b   Survivors of the atomic bomb explosions in Japan have had a statistically significant increase of leukemia as a function of their dose.
c   The National Academy of Sciences' "Biological Effects of Ionizing Radiation," 1972 (BEIR report) states that if all the population of the United States were to receive an additional 5 rems in 30 years, then roughly 3,000 to 15,000 cancer deaths annually would occur, depending on the assumptions used in the calculations.

Embryological Effect

The developing mammalian embryo, especially during its early development, is extremely sensitive to ionizing radiation.

A mammalian pregnancy is divided into three major periods:

1   Preimplantation
2   Major organogenesis
3   Fetus

The preimplantation period is when the fertilized egg or zygote is passing through the fallopian tube and has not yet been implanted in the uterus. This period in the human is approximately 8 to 10 days. The major organogenesis period is when the major organs of the body are being developed. In the human this period is approximately 6 to 7 weeks. The period of the fetus is when the organs of the mammal are being completed to a stage which will enable the mammal to survive after birth.

Figure 3-2 describes the effect of a single exposure of 200 R to mice as a function of the period of pregnancy.

If the single exposure of 200 R is delivered during the preimplantation stage, as high as 80 percent of the embryos die long before term. Note the

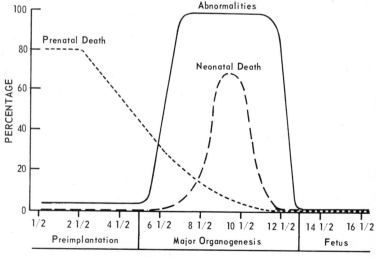

Figure 3-2 Effect of 200 R (single exposure) at different periods of mouse prenatal development. [L. B. Russell and W. L. Russell, *J. Cell and Comp. Physiol. Suppl.*, 1:43 (1954) (*Courtesy, The Wistar Press*).]

gradual decrease of prenatal deaths as the time of the single irradiation is delayed, until, if it were given at day fourteen (start of the period of the fetus in the mouse), the number of prenatal deaths would approach zero.

If the single exposure of 200 R is delivered during the period of major organogenesis, 100 percent of the embryos have abnormalities, with a high percentage of various skeletal and central nervous system malformations. Many of these abnormalities are too severe to be compatible with life, as can be seen by the large percentage of neonatal deaths (deaths of the fetus at about term).

If the single exposure of 200 R is delivered during the period of the fetus, the number of either abnormalities or neonatal deaths approaches zero. This illustrates the fact that the fetus is much more radioresistant than the developing embryo during the preimplantation or major organogenesis periods.

The previous chapter stated that the central nervous system (CNS) *after birth* is among the most radioresistant organ systems. However, during the early developing periods of the embryo (preimplantation and major organogenesis), it is among the most sensitive to ionizing radiation. This extreme radio-sensitivity of the developing CNS has been reported by researchers who have noted an effect on mammalian learning as a result of exposures as low as 25 R when given during the preimplantation period. Other animal experiments have shown that a dose of 10 rads to the embryo may produce deleterious effects. A United Nations report[9] linked radiation to retardation. In this human study, the dose from the atomic bombs dropped on Japan in 1945 ranged from 50 to 200 or more rads. Of the pregnant women who received 200 or more rads, 36 percent of the children were mentally retarded. To those who received 50 to 99 rads, 4.55 percent were mentally retarded. The report stated that a control population had less than a 1 percent rate of mentally retarded children.

Because of possible deleterious effects of ionizing radiation on the developing embryo, prior to a radiology procedure involving the abdomen of women of childbearing age, it is important for a practitioner to ascertain if she is pregnant and if so, the period of pregnancy. The practitioner can then decide as to whether or not the procedure should be immediately undertaken, postponed until later in the pregnancy, or postponed until after term.

Cataractogenic Effects

The lens of the eye focuses light on the retina in a manner similar to the lens of a camera. The fibers, which make up the lens are transparent to visible light. Ionizing radiation in large doses can damage these fibers as well as the immature cells which develop them. These damaged fibers are not as transparent to visible light, which results in decreased vision.

The sensitivity to radiation-induced cataracts is species dependent. Experiments have indicated that 10 to 30 rads will induce a cataract in the mouse. Information concerning radiation-induced cataracts in humans was obtained from the accidental exposure to the eyes of a relatively small number of workers. Investigations of these accidents indicated that a dose of 100 rads or more induced the cataracts. The eyes are considered a *critical organ* in terms of radiation protection, and as such the maximum permissible dose for radiation workers' eyes has been set at the same level as the whole body.

Life-Span Shortening

A decrease in the *average* life span as a function of a large radiation dose to a laboratory animal has been verified. It is important to understand that even if an animal has received a large dose of radiation, it does not mean that *that* animal will die sooner. However, if *all* the animals in a large colony received a large quantity of radiation, the average life of the animals would decrease statistically.

No unique diseases are produced as a function of radiation dose to cause average life-span shortening. Instead, a pattern of nonspecific life shortening is noted; i.e., the irradiated animals develop the same diseases as the nonirradiated ones, only sooner.

Figure 3-3 describes nonspecific life-span shortening. It depicts a hypothetical individual's life profile in terms of expected diseases.

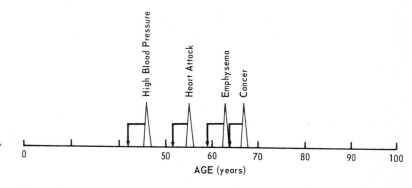

Figure 3-3 Example of nonspecific life-span shortening.

At a certain age, the hypothetical individual will develop high blood pressure, later he will suffer a heart attack, etc. Animal experiments have indicated that the onset of these diseases will be advanced as a function of radiation dose and that the diseases will be developed in the same sequence, only sooner. The mechanism of this effect is not well understood. It may be due, among other reasons, to errors induced by radiation in DNA coding or to capillary damage which causes decreased capillary flow, resulting in a decreased exchange of nutrients, oxygen, and waste materials from cells.

An experiment by Hursh[16] on rats and mice indicated that their life span was shortened 2.5 to 5 percent per 100 R after a single sublethal whole-body exposure. Other experiments by Moe[17] indicated that if the exposures to mice or guinea pigs were very small, their average life span was increased. Further studies are continuing on the question of the effect on the average life span by very low doses of ionizing radiation.

Retrospective studies in the United States indicate that the early radiologists (those who practiced during the early years of radiology) had an average decreased life span of approximately 5 years when compared with other physicians of the same time period. At the present time, the average life span of radiologists and other medical practitioners appears to be approximately the same.

COMMENT

There is a great benefit from the proper use of ionizing radiation in the healing arts. When ionizing radiation is judiciously used, the somatic risk to any individual is extremely minute. Therefore, do not be afraid of ionizing radiation, but respect it such that the maximum benefit is received with a minimum of exposure to all concerned.

QUESTIONS

3-1   Will a dose of 50 rads cause a decreased life span to an individual?
3-2   List four possible long-term somatic effects from excessive ionizing radiation.
3-3   Using a curvilinear model of dose response, if you double the dose will the response also be doubled?
3-4   Would you expect the prenatal deaths in mice from a single dose of 200 rads to decrease as a function of later exposure during pregnancy?
3-5   Why is the period of the fetus relatively radio-insensitive?

3-6   You are informed by a patient that she did not tell her physician she is 4 weeks pregnant and you find it necessary to repeat a KUB procedure. What would you do?

3-7   What is the relative radio-sensitivity of the central nervous system prior to birth? After birth?

3-8   What was a major long-term cause of death among radium-dial painters? Why?

3-9   Would you expect a study of radiologic technologists to show a cancer mortality rate which is essentially the same as that of the United States public?

3-10   Why is radium concentrated by the body in bone?

REFERENCES

1   Bacq, Z. M., and P. Alexander: "Fundamentals of Radiology," Pergamon, New York, 1961.

2   "The Effects on Populations of Exposure to Low Levels of Ionizing Radiation," Report of the Advisory Committee on the Biological Effects of Ionizing Radiation, National Academy of Sciences, National Research Council, Washington, D.C., 1972.

3   Laws, P. W.: "Medical and Dental X-rays—A Consumers Guide to Avoiding Unnecessary Radiation Exposure," Public Citizen, Health Research Group, Washington, D.C., 1974.

4   Yamazaki, J.: A Review of the Literature on the Radiation Dosage Required to Cause Manifest Central Nervous System Disturbances From In Utero and Post-natal Exposure, *Pediatrics,* vol. 37, no. 5, part II, May 1966.

5   De Groot, I. M. and Paloyan: Thyroid Carcinoma and Radiation—A Chicago Endemic, *JAMA,* vol. 225, no. 5, July 30, 1973.

6   Oman, R. M.: "An Introduction to Radiologic Science," McGraw-Hill, New York, 1975.

7   March: Leukemia in Radiologists, Ten Years Later, *Am. J. of the Medical Sciences,* Aug. 1961.

8   Lewis, E. B.: "Leukemia, Multiple Myeloma and Aplastic Anemia in American Radiologists," *Science,* Dec. 13, 1963.

9   *Report of the United Nations Scientific Committee on the Effects of Atomic Radiation,* General Assembly, Official Records: 24th Session, Supplement No. 13 (A/7613), 1969.

10   Barnett, Mark: "Biological Effects of Ionizing Radiation," U.S. Public Health Service, BRH, FDA Training Publication TP-37.

11   Schulz, R. J.: "Primer of Radiobiology," GAF Corporation, GAF Publication 6540-009, 1971.

12   *Report of the United Nations Scientific Committee on the Effects of Atomic Radiation,* United Nations, New York, 1962.

13   Glass, R.: "Mortality of New England Dentists, 1921-1960," Publication No. 999-RH-18, Washington, D.C., 1966.

14 Pifer, and Hemplemann: Radiation Induced Thyroid Carcinoma, *Annals of the New York Academy of Science,* vol. 114, pp. 838–848, April 2, 1964.
15 Rugh, R.: Ionizing Radiations and Congenital Anomalies of the Nervous System, *Mil. Med.,* vol. 127, pp. 883–907, Nov. 1962.
16 Hursh, J. B.: University of Rochester Report No. 506, Oct. 1957.
17 Moe, R.: *Nature,* vol. 180, p. 456, 1957.
18 NCRP: Review of the Current State of Radiation Protection Philosophy, *NCRP Report* 43, 1975.

Chapter 4

Biological Effects of Ionizing Radiation— Long-Term Genetic Effects

Objectives

The student learns about the possible long-term genetic implications of go-nad exposure to ionizing radiation. The student should

1   Be able to describe DNA base combinations and replication
2   Grasp the principle of DNA-RNA information coding
3   Understand the relationship of DNA-RNA gene expression
4   Appreciate the concept that most mutations produced by ionizing radiation are recessive

INTRODUCTION

The previous chapter discussed possible long-term somatic effects of ionizing radiation. This chapter will be concerned with possible long-term genetic (biological) effects which may not become manifest for years or even centuries following exposure.

The ability of humans to communicate concepts and skills through writing is truly remarkable. The English language has 26 letters, which form hundreds of thousands of words ranging in length from one letter to over twenty. In addition, there is a mathematical number component from zero to infinity as well as negative and imaginary numbers.

If it were ever possible to create the "blueprints" for a human being using the remarkable writing skills of language, it would no doubt take *many* volumes of books, illustrations, and narrative discussion. However, all this blueprint or genetic information is found in the nucleus of all the cells of your body with the exception of the mature erythrocytes (red blood cells).

The genetically active part of the genes in the chromosomes of the cell nucleus is actually deoxyribonucleic acid, or DNA. What makes this concept fascinating is that there is also a "written" language or code for DNA duplication leading to gene expression. However, unlike the alphabet, our DNA code has only *four* basic letters. A fifth letter is used for one stage of information coding transfer.

Also, our DNA (genes) do not have hundreds of thousands of words of virtually any letter length to choose from. Instead, they only have 64 possible words, of which there are only 20 meanings. Additionally, the words are all of the same length, three letters. With this information, we will develop the basic concepts of DNA replication and gene expression which the author hopes will illustrate some of the beauty, complexity, yet simplicity of nature and life.

BASIC DNA-RNA GENE EXPRESSION INTERACTIONS
DNA Base Combinations and Replication

The message or blueprint for a particular gene expression is found in the DNA. As stated above there are four basic letters in the genetic alphabet. These are four organic bases, two of which are chemically known as purines and two as pyrimidines.

Purines		Pyrimidines	
Adenine	(A)	Thymine	(T)
Guanine	(G)	Cytosine	(C)

For the purposes of this discussion we will call these four organic bases by the letters A, G, T, and C. Two of these letters in combination form each of the interconnections or "rungs" of the DNA rope ladder concept described in Chap. 2.

If a chemical organic model is made of each of these four letters and the models rotated through all possible angles, it would be noted that adenine will "fit" into thymine; that is, *A* would be able to join with *T*. However *A* would not fit into *G* or *C*. Therefore, the only possible combinations of adenine and thymine are *A-T* or *T-A*.

Rotation of the guanine *(G)* and cytosine *(C)* organic models indicates that they can "fit" only into each other, *G-C* or *C-G*, but that they cannot be joined with either *T* or *A*.

Therefore, the only possible combinations of the four organic base letters are

T-A	*G-C*
or	
A-T	*C-G*

T is a complement of *A* and vice versa. *G* is a complement of *C* and vice versa. This concept is illustrated in Fig. 4-1. The double-stranded DNA molecule is indicated as number 1 in the illustration. An enzyme causes the DNA molecule to cleave longitudinally, similar to the unzipping of a zipper (2 and 2*a*).

Each separated half of the DNA molecule has only one letter attached per interconnection of the former DNA rope ladder (2*b*). Within the nucleus of the cell, there are sizable quantities of nucleotides. Nucleotides are the organic base letters (*A, T, G,* and *C*) attached to a sugar-phosphate base. They can combine with the complementary letter on the single strand of DNA. As was discussed, *T* will combine with *A, G* with *C, A* with *T, C* with *G,* etc., to form the other half of the double-stranded DNA molecule (2*c*).

This occurs on each of the separated halves of the "unzipped" molecule resulting in two complete DNA molecules or chromosomes which are exact copies of each other (3). *This process occurs whenever the cell divides and results in two daughter cells which are genetically identical.*

Information Coding: DNA-RNA

This section will discuss the method by which the information or blueprint found in the DNA is translated into proteins.

As stated earlier, the DNA code is based on four basic letters, which form words only three letters long (triplets) with 20 usable meanings. In Fig. 4-2, the DNA has been unzipped by an enzyme to expose only one strand (*A*).

The words in DNA are triplets. The first triplet shown is *CAC,* followed by *GGC,* etc.

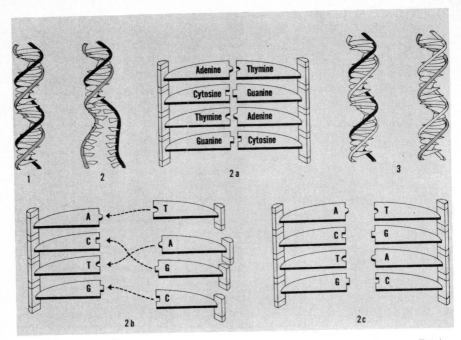

Figure 4-1 DNA base combinations and replication. (*Ward's Natural Science Establishment, Inc.*)

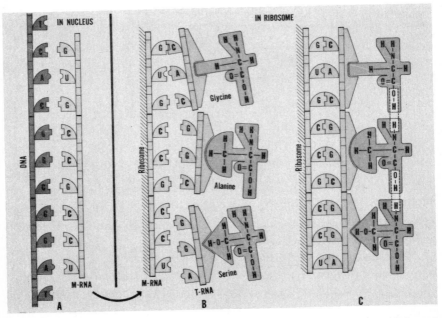

Figure 4-2 Information coding: DNA-RNA. (*Ward's Natural Science Establishment, Inc.*)

The single strand of DNA serves as a template upon which nucleotides are added to form *messenger ribonucleic acid* (mRNA). That is, *G* will combine with *C*, the first letter in the first word *CAC*. The second letter of the word is *A*. In mRNA the letter that combines with *A* is not *T*, but uracil *(U)*. Uracil is chemically similar to thymine and is the fifth letter of the DNA code discussed earlier in the chapter. The next letter of the DNA word *CAC* is *C*. The complementary letter to *C* is *G*, which is also formed on the mRNA. The mRNA now has the word *GUG*, which is the complement of the first DNA word *CAC*. This continues until the entire message in the particular gene has been copied. An enzyme then splits the mRNA away from the DNA. It can then leave the nucleus, migrate to the cytoplasm of the cell, and become affixed to a ribosome (B). In the ribosome, a second type of RNA known as transfer RNA (tRNA) is available. Each tRNA is a triplet which is a single word.

There are 64 possible combinations of triplet words from the four available letters. Some of these words appear to be meaningless while others are equivalent to punctuation; i.e., they tell when a particular word sequence has been completed. Of the remaining words, there are 20 different meanings. Some of the triplets, although spelled differently, have the same meaning.

If an organic model is made of the first triplet in Fig. 4-2 *(CAC)*, it is found that one and only one specific amino acid (glycine) can "fit." Therefore, only glycine will be affixed to the tRNA word *CAC*.

The amino acid alanine, and only alanine, can fit into and become attached to the next triplet word *GGU*. Each of the 20 basic amino acids has specific triplet words to which they, and only they, can be affixed. Therefore, the 20 words of the DNA vocabulary translate into the 20 basic amino acids.

The first word in the above DNA message, *CAC*, translates into commanding the ribosomes to place the amino acid glycine in a specific location. The next word of DNA, *GGC*, translates into placing the amino acid alanine next to the glycine. This process continues until the entire word message of the DNA gene is translated into placing specific amino acids in prespecified locations alongside the mRNA.

As the alignment of the amino acids is completed, a water molecule is split off (C) so that the amino acids join to form a protein. Proteins are long-chain amino acids formed in a specific order. Hair is a protein, as is insulin, but they are not identical since the amino acids are not in the same identical arrangement. If even one amino acid is out of place, the characteristics of the protein can be changed.

The basic function of DNA, then, is to tell the ribosome how to construct specific proteins. Proteins are essential for life and are a major component of many body structures, as well as hormones and enzymes.

DNA-RNA Gene Expression

As discussed in the previous section, the genetic coding message is transferred from the DNA to the ribosomes. The ribosomes then synthesize specific proteins by assembling the amino acids according to the programmed instructions of DNA. This is sequentially shown as numbers 1a, 1b, 2b, and 2c in Fig. 4-3.

Certain proteins can combine with a vitamin (3e) to form an enzyme (3f). An enzyme is an organic catalyst which modifies the rate of chemical reactions.

A specific enzyme causes a chemical reaction to occur. In the case of Fig. 4-3, black pigment is synthesized (4) which manifests itself as the gene expression (5), black hair on the rabbit.

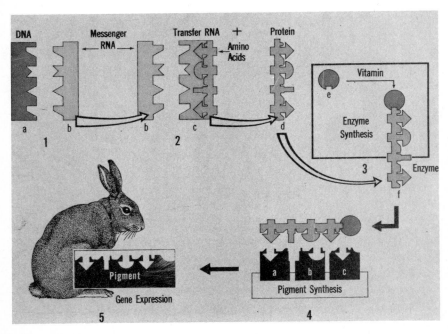

Figure 4-3 DNA-RNA gene expression. (*Ward's Natural Science Establishment, Inc.*)

Therefore, the original message for black hair was carried from DNA, to RNA, to the synthesis of a protein, to the combination of the protein with a vitamin to form an enzyme, to pigment synthesis resulting in black hair.

These gene messages from DNA which manifest themselves as a specific active gene expression are known as *dominant* genes. They produce an enzyme that causes a specific effect to occur.

If the programmed message is changed by as little as one letter in the original DNA code, a different protein could be synthesized which in combination with a vitamin may produce an enzyme that does not work. The gene that contains the modified coding is called *recessive* in that unlike a dominant gene, it does not lead to the synthesis of an enzyme which causes a specific effect to occur. If an individual has two recessive genes for the same trait, then the characteristic of the body without the modifying factors of enzymes to cause a specific effect will manifest itself. An example of this condition is albinism. If the individual has both a dominant and a recessive gene for the same trait, the trait may manifest itself fully or, depending upon the trait characteristics, in a modified form.

We all carry numerous mutations or recessive traits in our gene pool. Nature has been able to establish an equilibrium insofar as deleterious mutations are concerned by the process of survival of the fittest. Medical science is altering this balance by improved techniques to overcome many inherited deleterious conditions.

IONIZING-RADIATION EFFECTS

DNA Modification

Ionizing radiation can induce point mutations in DNA. This can result in one or more of the base coding letters being removed from the DNA. If this occurs, there will be a change in coding instructions which causes a modification of the enzyme protein. The new enzyme may not work, which means that a recessive mutation has occurred following exposure to ionizing radiation. Although it is conceivable that some of the mutations induced by ionizing radiation may result in a new enzyme that does cause a specific trait to become manifest (therefore, a dominant gene mutation), the majority of mutations have been found to be recessive.

The recessive traits induced by ionizing radiation do not become fully apparent until an individual is conceived who carries both recessive genes of the same trait. It thus may take many generations before the harmful effects of radiation exposure of the reproductive organs are observable.

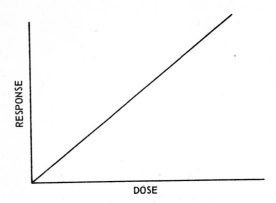

Figure 4-4 Linear dose-response curve.

Dose-Effect

In terms of the dose-effect relationship, a linear hypothesis, as illustrated in Fig. 4-4, is suggested for the genetic effect of ionizing radiation.

Since the linear dose-effect concept has no threshold (a dose below which there is no effect), it is important to minimize human exposure to all nonproductive ionizing radiation. The use of gonad shields, as appropriate, is of paramount importance in minimizing exposure to the reproductive organs. The possible long-term genetic effects of ionizing radiation form part of the basis for the maximum permissible dose equivalents for both occupationally and non-occupationally exposed individuals. This is discussed in the next chapter.

QUESTIONS

4-1   What are the basic letters of the DNA code? List which letters are complementary to each other.

4-2   Why are there only 20 basic meanings in the DNA code?

4-3   How is the message of DNA transferred to the ribosomes?

4-4   What is the function of the ribosomes?

4-5   What determines if a gene is dominant or recessive?

4-6   Why are we, in terms of radiation protection, so concerned about the possible long-term genetic effects of ionizing radiation?

4-7   Describe what can happen to a gene when it is exposed to ionizing radiation.

4-8   Discuss, in terms of radiation protection implications, the no-threshold concept of the linear genetic dose-response curve.

4-9   What is the function of tRNA?

4-10 What are nucleotides? Describe their function.

REFERENCES

1 Kirk, D.: "Biology Today," 2d ed., Random House, New York, 1975.
2 NCRP: Review of the Current State of Radiation Protection Philosophy, *NCRP Report* 43, 1975.
3 Cairns, J.: The Bacterial Chromosome, *Scientific American,* January 1966.
4 Bacq, Z. M., and P. Alexander: "Fundamentals of Radiobiology," Pergamon, New York, 1961.
5 "The Effects on Populations of Exposure to Low Levels of Ionizing Radiation," National Academy of Sciences, National Research Council, November 1972.

Chapter 5

Maximum Permissible Dose Equivalents (MPD)

Objectives

The student learns about the basic concepts of maximum permissible dose equivalents both for radiation workers and the general public. The student should

1 Comprehend the basic radiation protection philsophy
2 Know the maximum permissible dose equivalents (MPD) for radiation workers
3 Realize how to calculate maximum permissible dose equivalents allowed to occupationally exposed individuals per calendar quarter for radiation
4 Understand emergency exposure concepts
5 Have knowledge about the maximum permissible dose equivalents for the non-occupationally exposed public

BASIC RADIATION PROTECTION PHILOSOPHY

One of the questions most frequently asked by both radiation workers and the general public is, "How much radiation can I receive and still be safe from any adverse effects?"

In order to answer this question, we must discuss two of the current concepts of radiation dose-response curves. One possible type of response can be seen in the curve in Fig. 5-1.

Note that as the dose decreases, the response also decreases until a point is reached where there is *no* response. This point is known as the *threshold,* i.e., a point below which radiation will elicit no response. This S-shaped dose-response curve is known as a sigmoid curve. Many types of somatic responses to radiation appear to follow this sigmoid curve, e.g., death, erythema, epilation, etc.

Another possible dose-response curve is shown as Fig. 5-2.

Here the response also decreases as a function of dose, but there is no threshold; i.e., there is no dose below which there is no response. This linear (straight-line) curve appears to be the correct mode of dose-response for genetic effects and for certain somatic effects (e.g., leukemia).

The correct curve (or combination of the two curves) for the low-dose, low-energy radiation typically found in the practice of radiologic technology is still the subject of intensive investigation and controversy. However, the National Council on Radiation Protection and Measurements (NCRP) states, "The most important radiation health hazards do not have a dose threshold. On this basis, the setting of radiation protection standards re-

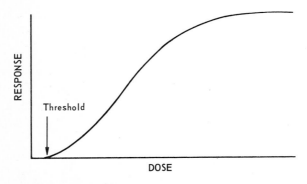

Figure 5-1 Sigmoid dose-response curve.

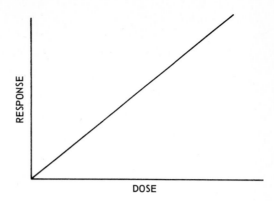

Figure 5-2 Linear dose-response curve.

quires consideration of compensatory trade-offs between currently assumed hazards and benefits."*

The Environmental Protection Agency (EPA), Office of Radiation Programs, issued a policy statement (March 3, 1975) which also assumed for purpose of estimating potential health impact, that there is a linear, nonthreshold relationship between the magnitude of the radiation dose received and effect.

By assuming the linear nonthreshold curve, the reader can ascertain that there is *no* level of radiation below which the individual is absolutely safe. However, based on risk assumptions published by the International Commission on Radiological Protection (ICRP) and other scientifically renowned organizations, the probability of any adverse effects to an individual whose dose is kept under the guidelines below will be exceedingly remote.

The maximum permissible dose equivalents as developed in this chapter should be considered only as upper limits which should not be exceeded without careful consideration of the reasons for doing so; all exposures should be kept to a practicable minimum. From this philsophy, the question as to how much radiation is safe can be answered by responding that, on the conservative assumption that there is no threshold, every use of radiation potentially involves a small risk but that use of radiation in the healing arts results in such numerous benefits that if judiciously used the benefits of radiation greatly exceed the very small risk to the individual.

* NCRP, Review of the Current State of Radiation Protection Philosophy, *NCRP Report* 43, p. 2, 1975.

Maximum permissible dose equivalents (MPDs) are divided into two major categories: occupationally exposed (radiation worker), and non-occupationally exposed (general public). These standards are for radiation exposures received from other than natural background radiation and the healing arts use of radiation. Therefore, a radiation worker who, as a patient, requires radiation for the diagnosis or treatment of disease should remove his personnel dosimeter (i.e., film badge) before the procedure begins.

RADIATION WORKERS

Prospective Annual Limit

The United Nations Scientific Committee on the Effects of Atomic Radiation (UNSCEAR) issued a report in 1972 updating earlier estimates of genetic risks. The report estimated that, depending upon dose rate, the doubling dose for the mouse for genetic mutations was somewhere between 16 and 100 rems. The doubling dose is that quantity of radiation which would double the natural genetic mutation rate.

An individual is not expected to become a radiation worker until age 18. In addition, the great majority of children are conceived prior to their parents' reaching age 30, a time frame for the radiation worker of 12 years $(30 - 18 = 12)$.

Radiation workers, taking into account their 12 working years until age 30, may receive a dose equivalent of 60 rems to the gonads. This may be, for radiation protection purposes, considered a doubling dose. If 60 rems may be received in 12 years, then the average per year is

$$\frac{60 \text{ rems}}{12 \text{ years}} = 5 \text{ rems per year, or 5,000 mrens per year}$$

If one assumes a working year of 50 weeks, then the average weekly dose equivalent would be

$$\frac{5,000 \text{ mrems per year}}{50 \text{ weeks per year}} = 100 \text{ mrems per week}$$

Therefore 100 mrems per week average may be considered as the gonad maximum permissible dose equivalent (MPD) for occupational exposure and is also the MPD for exposure of the whole body, blood-forming organs, and lens of eye, for occupationally exposed workers.

Because radiation workers may receive partial body exposure, special maximum permissible dose equivalents for skin, hands, forearms, and other organs have been established. These are summarized below in Table 5-1.

In addition, because of the increased sensitivity of the developing fetus, the NCRP and the U.S. Nuclear Regulatory Commission (NRC, formerly the Atomic Energy Commission) have suggested guidelines with respect to the fetus for occupational exposure to pregnant women. It is recommended that "during the entire gestation period, the maximum permissible dose equivalent to the fetus from occupational exposures of the expectant mother should not exceed 0.5 rem."*

Retrospective Annual Occupational Dose Equivalent

As discussed earlier, a radiation worker may receive, on the average, a maximum dose equivalent of 5.0 rems per year.

In addition, the current guidelines state that he may receive a retrospective annual occupational dose equivalent of 3 rems per calendar quarter, or 12 rems per year—*if* he has the rems in what we will call "a rem bank account."

The maximum possible long-term accumulation of combined whole-body dose equivalent (assessed in the gonads, lens of the eye, or red bone marrow) can be calculated on the basis of 5 rems per year starting at age 18, that is, the maximum accumulative dose equivalent is equal to $5(N-18)$ where N is the age in years.

Problem   What is the maximum number of rems a radiation worker can have received by age 25?

Answer

$$5(N - 18)$$
$$N = \text{age} = 25 \text{ years}$$

Therefore the maximum number of rems the radiation worker could have received is

$$5(25 - 18) = 5(7) = 35 \text{ rems}$$

We then subtract from the 35 rems the known occupationally received rems from age 18, to obtain what we will call his current rem bank account.

* NCRP, Basic Radiation Protection, *NCRP Report* 39, p. 92, 1971.

Problem If through personnel dosimeter records it is ascertained that the above worker has received 7 rems since age 18, what is his rem bank account?

Answer

$$35 \text{ rems} - 7 \text{ rems} = 28 \text{ rems}$$

Problem As discussed earlier in this section, the radiation worker can receive 12 rems per year *if* he has the rems in his rem bank account. Can this worker receive 12 rems in the next year of work?

Answer Yes, he has 28 rems in the rem bank account at the beginning of the year, plus accumulating 5 additional rems during the year for a total of 33 rems. We can then subtract the 12 rems dose equivalent received during the year to leave a total of 21 rems remaining in his rem bank account.

Special Situations

Students The case of students who are less than 18 years old presents a special situation. The NCRP recommends that these students should not receive a whole-body dose equivalent exceeding 0.1 rem per year due to their

Table 5-1 Maximum Permissible Dose Equivalents for Occupational Exposure

Combined whole body	
Prospective annual limit	5 rems per year
Retrospective annual limit	12 rems per year
Long-term accumulation	$5(N - 18)$ where N is the age in years
Skin	15 rems per year
Forearms	30 rems per year (10 rems per quarter)
Hands	75 rems per year (25 rems per quarter)
Other organs, tissues, and organ systems	15 rems per year (5 rems per quarter)
Fertile women (with respect to the fetus)	0.5 rem in gestation period
Special situations	
Students under age 18	0.1 rem per year
Emergency dose limits—life saving	
Individuals (older than 45 if possible)	100 rems
Hands and forearms	200 rems, additional (300 rems, total)
Emergency dose limits—less urgent	
Individual	25 rems
Hands and forearms	100 rems, total

educational activity.* It is the responsibility of the educational institution to monitor carefully those students using personnel dosimeters. When the student becomes 18 years old, then he is an occupational worker and is subject to the maximum dose equivalents previously discussed, that is, 5.0 rem per year average.

Emergency Situations   In the highly unlikely event of exposure received by a radiation worker during the course of a life-saving action of less urgent emergency, dose limits cannot be specified. However, the recommendations listed in Table 5-1 for such situations are listed as guidelines.†

NON-OCCUPATIONALLY EXPOSED (GENERAL PUBLIC)
General Concepts

Human beings from their earliest existence have lived in a sea of radiation emitted from the sun, the stars, and the earth itself. This natural background of radiation varies as a function of different locations on the earth as well as other environmental factors. It is estimated that the average gonad dose equivalent in the United States from natural background radiation is 88 mrem per year.‡ The human race has demonstrated an ability to survive in spite of any adverse effects from this quantity of radiation. However, in order to minimize any possible deleterious effects from additional sources of radiation, it is prudent and reasonable to establish guidelines for the general public. These guidelines are exclusive of natural background radiation and healing arts radiation received by the general public for diagnosis or treatment.

In 1957 the NCRP recommended that the maximum dose to individuals in the general population should be limited to one-tenth of the occupational level for whole body, head, trunk, active blood-forming organs, or gonads. Since the occupational MPD is 5.0 rems per year, the MPD for *an individual* in the general population for the whole body or organs listed above is 0.5 rem per year. This same limit was adapted by the Federal Radiation Council (FRC) in 1960 and reaffirmed by the NCRP in 1975.

The FRC as well as the NCRP recommends that the *average* general population dose equivalent from man-made radiation (again, exclusive of

* NCRP, Radiation Protection in Educational Institutions, *NCRP Report* 32, p. 8, 1966.
† *NCRP Report* 39 (1971) should be consulted for more complete information on emergency guidelines.
‡ Natural Radiation Exposure in the United States, EPA, ORP/SID 72-1, p. 38, 1972.

Table 5-2   Maximum Permissible Dose Equivalents for the Public

Individual	0.5 rem per year
Genetic—average	0.17 rem per year. *Average*
Somatic—average	0.17 rem per year. *Average*
Family of Radioactive Patients	
Individual (under age 45)	0.5 rem per year
Individual (over age 45)	5.0 rems per year

healing arts or natural background radiation) be limited to 5 rems in 30 years or 5 rems/30 years = 0.167 rem per year.

A special exception is made for the family of radioactive patients. These patients have either had radioactive implants or organ uptake of radioactive materials. The NCRP recommends that individuals (under age 45) of such families be limited to 0.5 rem in any one year, while those over age 45 may receive as much as 5 rems in one year.

Table 5-2 below summarizes the maximum permissible dose equivalents recommended for the public.

State Regulations

Many states have regulatory maximum permissible dose equivalents which may not be identical with these national guidelines. Therefore, the reader is requested to contact his respective state radiation control program for additional information (see listing in Appendix).

QUESTIONS

5-1   What is the maximum dose equivalent per year (MPD) for whole-body exposure for radiologic technology students over age 18?

5-2   What is the maximum dose equivalent per year (MPD) for whole-body exposure for radiologic technology students under age 18?

5-3   What action(s) would you recommend if a radiologic technologist student under age 18 approaches the yearly MPD? Why?

5-4   Why can the MPDs for radiologic technologists (radiation workers) be virtually a doubling dose of radiation, while the general public MPD is only a small fraction of a possible doubling dose of radiation?

5-5   What is the maximum allowable dose equivalent a radiation worker may have received who is 21 years old?

5-6   If the radiation worker in Prob. 5-5 has received a total dose equivalent of 7 rems, can he receive 12 rems during the next work year? During the second year? Explain your answer.

5-7   What actions would you take, as a supervisor, if a radiologic technologist's film badge read 85 mR in one month, while most technologists' badges read less than 20 mR per month? Is the 85 mR per month reading dangerous?

5-8   For radiation protection purposes, how much may an individual of the general population receive per year from man-made non-healing arts sources of radiation?

5-9   If a radiologic technologist receives radiation as a patient, does this count against his rem bank account?

5-10   What is the MPD (with respect to the fetus) of pregnant radiation workers? What actions would you take, as a supervisor, if a radiologic technologist informs you she is 4 months pregnant?

REFERENCES

1   NCRP: Review of the Current State of Radiation Protection Philosophy, *NCRP Report* 43, 1975.

2   Federal Radiation Council: Background Material for the Development of Radiation Protection Standards, FRC Report No. 1, 1960.

3   NCRP: Basic Radiation Protection Criteria, *NCRP Report* 39, 1971.

4   NCRP: Radiation Protection in Educational Institutions, *NCRP Report* 32, 1966.

5   U.S. Environmental Protection Agency: "Natural Radiation Exposure in the United States," U.S. Environmental Protection Agency, Rockville, Md., 1972.

6   International Commission on Radiological Protection: "The Evaluation of Risks from Radiation," ICRP Publications, Pergamon, London, 1968.

7   National Academy of Sciences–National Research Council: The Effects on Populations of Exposure to Low Levels of Ionizing Radiation, 1972.

8   United Nations Scientific Committee on the Effect of Atomic Radiation: Ionizing Radiation: Levels and Effects, United Nations, New York, 1972.

Chapter 6

Ionizing-Radiation
Detection Instruments

Objectives

The student learns the uses and limitations of the various types of instruments used in ionizing-radiation detection. The student should

1 Be aware of the two general classes of instruments used
2 Know how to describe the method of operation of personnel pocket chambers and self-reading dosimeters
3 Comprehend the method of detection and readout for both film badges and thermoluminescent dosimeters (TLD)
4 Understand the basic concepts of the limitations and use of field survey meters

In general, the various types of instruments used in the field by health physicists and/or radiologic technologists to detect ionizing radiation can be classified into two general categories: (1) personnel monitoring devices and (2) field survey instruments.

59

PERSONNEL MONITORING DEVICES

Pocket Dosimeters

Method of Operation   Pocket dosimeters consist basically of two electrodes, one positively charged and one negatively charged. The central electrode is insulated from the outer electrode, as illustrated in Fig. 6-1. Please note that part of the central electrode (anode) consists of a movable fiber.

Prior to use, the chamber is charged. Since like charges repel, the movable fiber pushes away from the central stationary electrodes, as shown in Fig. 6-1.

Ionizing radiation interacts with the air within the chamber or the walls of the chamber to form positively charged ions and negatively charged electrons. The electrons migrate to the central electrode (unlike charges attract) to form neutral atoms. Therefore, the number of positive ions within the central electrode is reduced as a function of the amount of radiation interacting in the air or walls of the chamber.

As the number of positive ions within the central electrode are reduced, the charge is also reduced. This means that the repelling force between the movable fiber and the stationary central electrode has also been reduced. The net result is that the movable fiber is now closer to the stationary central electrode. This concept is illustrated in Fig. 6-2.

By the use of special optics, we can calibrate on a viewable scale the

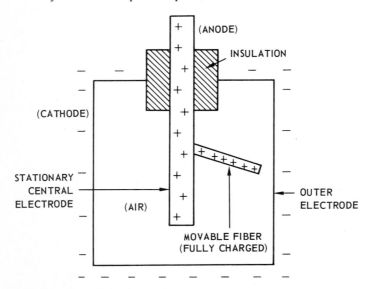

Figure 6-1   Charged electroscope.

distance the movable fiber is from the stationary central electrode versus exposure. With a maximum charge the scale will read zero. As the charge decreases, the reading on the viewable scale will increase. A typical example of the viewable scale is shown in Fig. 6-3.

The long vertical line (which in Fig. 6-3 reads approximately 70 mR) is actually the movable fiber. Remember, when it is fully charged, it is calibrated to read zero; as it discharges, the line will move toward the right indicating additional exposure.

The radiologic technologist can utilize this device *if* the walls of the chamber are essentially air equivalent* for the energy of the x-rays being

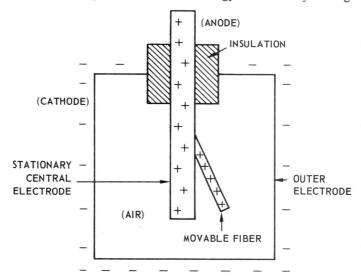

Figure 6-2 Partially discharged electroscope.

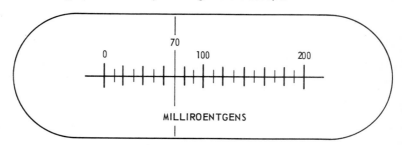

Figure 6-3 Pocket dosimeter—viewable scale.

* Air equivalent walls means that the effective Z number of the wall is essentially that of air.

used; in other words, if the chamber is classified as a *low-energy dosimeter* (LED). The technologist should not attempt to utilize a typical civil defense type of pocket dosimeter since it contains a metal wall which is not air equivalent so that erroneous readings could occur.

Using the low-energy dosimeter (LED) for diagnostic x-ray personnel monitoring, the technologist notes and records the initial reading of the pocket dosimeter. It does not have to read zero. At the end of the day (or procedure) he notes and records the final reading. The difference between the initial and final readings is the integrated exposure received by the dosimeter.

Since the electrical charge will eventually "leak off," the reading of the pocket dosimeter will increase as a function of time even though there has been no radiation exposure. Therefore, the wearer must take daily initial and final readings to approximate the exposure. In addition, if there is a dust accumulation of the contacts of the pocket dosimeter or a breakdown of the integrity of the insulation, there is a possibility of increased leakage of the charge so as to give a serious erroneous reading of exposure. There is also the possibility that a sudden shock (dropping it on the floor) will discharge the chamber resulting again in an erroneous reading of exposure.

In order to minimize any erroneous readings, it is recommended that the wearer utilize two pocket dosimeters and record the lower readings at the end of each day.

Types   There are two basic types of pocket dosimeters: (1) pocket chambers and (2) self-reading pocket dosimeters.

Pocket Chambers   The pocket chamber is an integrating device and requires a special charger-reader in order to be utilized. A typical pocket chamber is illustrated in Fig. 6-4.

The pocket chamber is read by inserting it into the charger-reader and viewing the scale through a special lens.

Self-Reading Pocket Dosimeter   The self-reading pocket dosimeter is charged in a similar manner as a pocket chamber by using a charger. However, by the use of a double convex lens, it can be immediately read by holding the dosimeter to a light and directly reading the scale.

The self-reading pocket dosimeter is more expensive than the pocket chamber but has the major advantage of being able to be read immediately by the radiologic technologist without inserting it into the charger-reader.

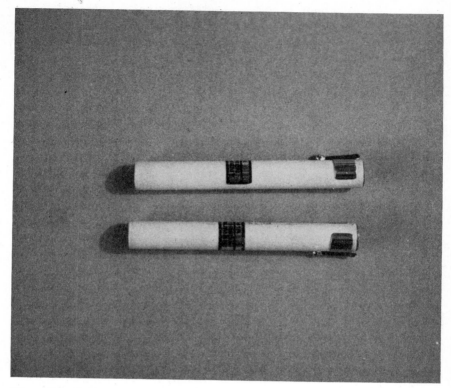

Figure 6-4 Pocket chamber.

Film Badges

The film badge is currently one of the most popular methods for personnel monitoring. A typical film badge is illustrated in Fig. 6-6.

The film badge consists of a clip-on holder with an open portion (window). In addition various filters of different metals are attached to the holder so that the ratio of the film densities under each of the filters can be made. This is required prior to interpretation of personnel exposure in order to determine the x-ray energy distribution. Although a detailed explanation of this requirement is beyond the planned scope of this text, suffice it to state that the density of film following exposure to x-rays is dependent not only on the quantity of radiation received, but also on the energy of the radiation. Therefore, the energy distribution of the x-ray field must be ascertained. Figure 6-7 shows the filters of a film badge.

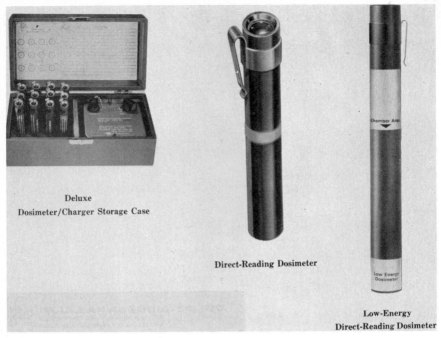

Figure 6-5 Self-reading dosimeters. (*Nuclear Associates, Inc.*)

Deluxe
Dosimeter/Charger Storage Case

Direct-Reading Dosimeter

Low-Energy
Direct-Reading Dosimeter

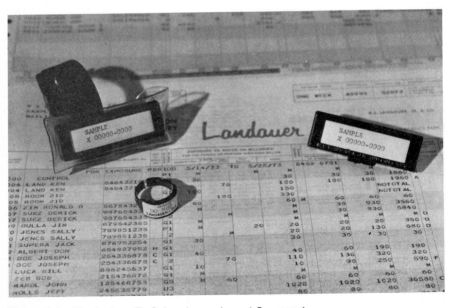

Figure 6-6 Film badge. (R. S. Landauer, Jr. and Company)

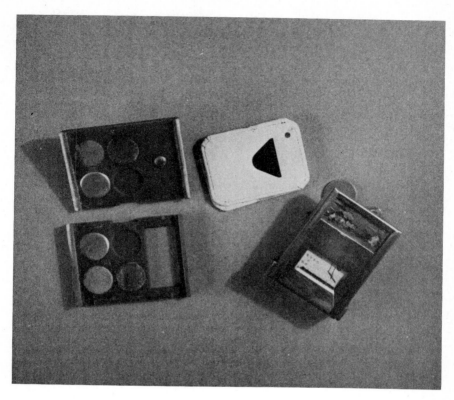

Figure 6-7 Film badge filters.

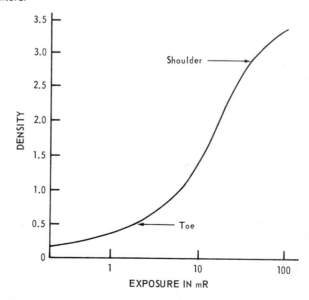

Figure 6-8 Typical characteristic curve.

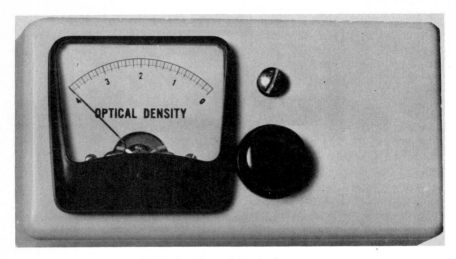

Figure 6-9 Densitometer. (*Nuclear Associates, Inc.*)

Once the x-ray energy distribution is determined by the use of filter–film-density ratios, a characteristic curve can be made using known exposures of the same x-ray energy distribution to film badges. A typical characteristic curve is shown in Fig. 6-8.

Following the development of a film badge, its density is determined by a densitometer. If by using the characteristic curve illustrated in Fig. 6-8 the density of the film badge in question is found to be 1.5, then the interpretation is that the film was exposed to 10 mR.

If the x-ray energy distribution to the film is correctly determined by the use of filter–film-density ratios, a film badge is capable of fairly accurate interpretations of exposure. In addition, the film badge has been used as a permanent legal record of exposure and is relatively inexpensive.

The main disadvantage of a film badge is that the wearer has to wait until the badge is processed for the dose to be determined. This means that by the time the film badge results are received the wearer may not recall the specific instances leading to any high exposures.

Thermoluminescent Dosimeters

A thermoluminescent dosimeter (TLD) may be similar in outward appearance to a film badge. A typical thermoluminescent dosimeter is illustrated in Fig. 6-10.

A TLD system consists of crystals which as a result of exposure to ionizing radiation undergo changes in certain of their physical properties.

Lithium fluoride (LiF) and manganese-activated calcium fluoride (CaF_2:Mn) are two crystals which can be used for TLDs used in diagnostic radiology.

As the reader recalls, an atom has specific electron orbits around the nucleus. The immediate area past the outermost or valence orbit is known as the forbidden-band region. Electrons are not normally found in the forbidden-band region. The next higher energy level where electrons can be normally found is the conduction band. Electrons in the conduction band are free to travel as in metal electrical conductors. A simplified example of this concept is shown in Fig. 6-11.

The solids commonly used in TLDs are crystals which contain defects in their lattice or crystalline structure caused either naturally or by the addition of an impurity.

The result of these defects permits electrons which are released from orbits, as a result of increased energy acquired from the interaction of ioniz-

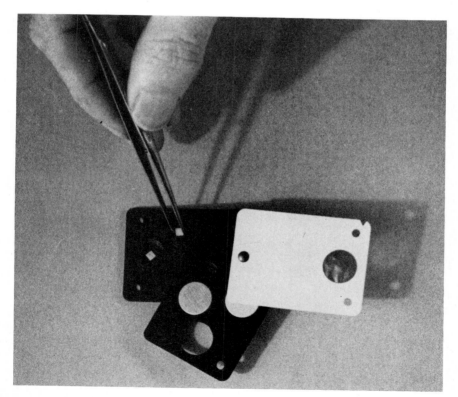

Figure 6-10 Thermoluminescent dosimeter.

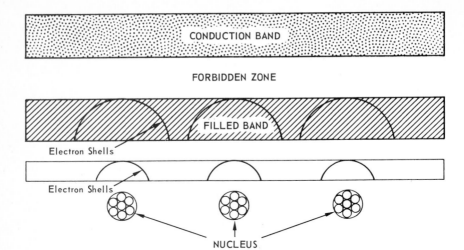

Figure 6-11 Electron energy levels.

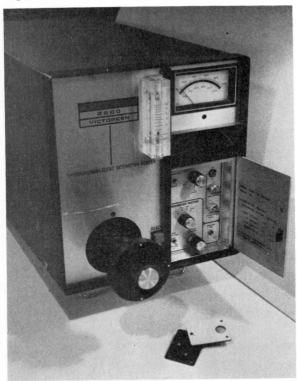

Figure 6-12 Thermoluminescent dosimeter reader. (*Victoreen Instrument Division.*)

ing radiation with matter, to become "trapped" in the forbidden-band region.

If the crystal were then heated, the electrons would acquire additional energy such that they would be freed from their trap and migrate up to the conduction band (where electrons are mobile and can travel), eventually returning to their normal position and emitting their excess energy in the form of a light photon.

Therefore, if we expose a TLD crystal to a known quantity of radiation and heat the crystal, a measurable quantity of light would be emitted. This light is quantitatively measured by a suitable readout instrument. Since the intensity of the light emitted from the TLD is directly proportional to the ionizing radiation received, it is possible to calibrate the light output to the radiation dose. In this way, a certain intensity of light flash could be correlated to a specific radiation dose.

Since, following the heating of the TLD, the electrons have returned to their normal positions, there is no permanent record other than the readout instrument recorder. The TLD following proper heating (annealing) can be used over again.

Certain TLDs may have a fading problem; i.e., the trapped electrons can, as a function of time, be slowly released from their traps to return to their normal position. This can lead to errors in dose assessment. For example, LiF has a fading rate of only about 5 percent per year while CaF_2:Mn has a fading rate of about 10 to 20 percent per month. Manganese-activated calcium sulfate ($CaSO_4$:Mn) is much more sensitive to ionizing radiation but has a fading rate as high as 50 percent in 24 h. An advantage of LiF and CaF_2:Mn is that they provide relatively accurate readings in the diagnostic x-ray range without the necessity of attempting to determine the x-ray energy distribution.

FIELD SURVEY INSTRUMENTS*

The Ionization Chamber Type

This type of survey instrument records x- or gamma radiation (or, with an appropriate window, beta radiation). A typical example is illustrated in Fig. 6-13. This instrument can be used as a *rate* meter (that is, mR/h) or, in

---

* Although the diagnostic radiologic technologist does not normally utilize field survey instruments in their daily professional activities, this section is presented for their general information and to acquaint them with the instrumentation in the event of their use. For questions pertaining to the specific use of instruments the radiologic technologist should contact either a health physicist or the institute radiation safety officer.

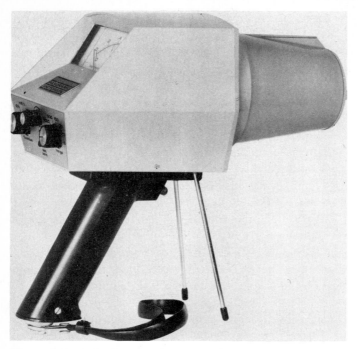

Figure 6-13 Ionization chamber survey instrument. (*Victoreen Instrument Division.*)

certain models, as an integrating device (total mR exposure). Some models are equipped with either removable or remotely attached ionization measuring chambers.

An advantage of this type of instrument is that it is relatively accurate in the diagnostic x-ray range (± 20 percent).

A disadvantage is the relatively long period of time it takes to reach the maximum meter reading. The meter reading will increase rapidly at first but can take several seconds to reach its maximum response. Therefore, unless the response time of the instrument is carefully taken into account, the brief time exposures typically found in diagnostic radiology will not be of sufficient duration to permit the meter to reach its maximum response. This can result in an erroneous low interpretation of the radiation field.

Geiger Counter

This instrument is used for recording x- or gamma radiation as well as for beta particle monitoring. A typical portable Geiger counter is shown in Fig. 6-14. Although the Geiger counter can be calibrated and used for x-ray

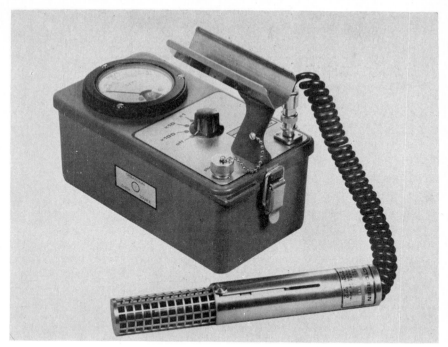

Figure 6-14 Geiger counter. (*Victoreen Instrument Division.*)

monitoring, it is normally calibrated for higher-energy gamma rays. Since, in most Geiger counters, the sensitive chamber is enclosed by a metal which is not air equivalent in the diagnostic x-ray range, the instrument (unless specifically calibrated) will not give the correct exposure rates. Therefore, unless the Geiger counter has a special probe sensitive to and calibrated in the diagnostic x-ray range, it *should not be used* for diagnostic x-ray surveys but limited in use to the rapid monitoring of contamination from radioactive materials or for gamma-ray measurements.

QUESTIONS

6-1 A radiologic technologist is utilizing two self-reading pocket dosimeters for personnel monitoring. At the end of the day, one dosimeter's integrated exposure reads 3 mR, while the other reads 84 mR. Which one of the two should the technologist record? Why?

6-2 Is it necessary for the pocket chamber (or self-reading pocket dosimeter) to read zero as an initial reading?

6-3 List several advantages and disadvantages of pocket dosimeters.

6-4   What is the major reason to have filters of various metals on film badges? Why
          is this so important?
6-5   List several advantages and disadvantages of film badges.
6-6   Explain the basic theory of thermoluminescent dosimetry.
6-7   List several advantages and disadvantages of TLDs.
6-8   What is meant by a rate meter? By an integrating device?
6-9   Should Geiger counters be used in diagnostic x-ray surveys or measurements?
          Why?
6-10 Can a typical ionization rate meter be used to determine actual exposure rates
          during radiographic examinations?

REFERENCES

1   Cember, H.: "Introduction to Health Physics," Pergamon, New York, 1969.
2   Oman, R.M.: "An Introduction to Radiologic Science," McGraw-Hill, New
        York, 1975.
3   Handloser, J. S.: "Health Physics Instrumentation," Pergamon, New York, 1956.
4   Moe, H. J. et al.: "Radiation Safety Technician Training Course Manual," ANL-
        7291, Rev. 1, National Technical Information Service, U.S. Department of Com-
        merce, 1972.

Chapter 7

Factors Affecting Radiographic Images

Objectives

The student acquires an understanding of the basic factors which affect radiographic images. The student should

1 Be aware of the principles of radiographic density and contrast
2 Be able to describe a characteristic curve
3 Understand both radiographic contrast and definition
4 Know two factors which affect radiographic contrast and definition
5 Be able to show how each of these factors affects radiographic images

REVIEW OF FUNDAMENTALS

Density

As light (or x-ray) photons interact with film, a latent image in the crystals of silver halide is formed. A latent image can be defined as the complex forma-

73

tion of several atoms of free silver in a silver halide crystal as a result of the interaction of photons or charged particles.

Since silver in the crystal is found as the positive ion (Ag^+) the initial interactions of radiation have caused several silver ions to be reduced; i.e., some of the electrons liberated as a result of interaction have combined with several silver ions to *reduce* the charge of the silver ions to zero, or neutral.

The film is then placed in a developer (an alkaline reducing agent) which differentially reduces (forms free silver) those crystals which have a latent image. This means that the free silver in those crystals that have a latent image act like a catalyst and are developed before the crystals that do not have any latent images. The net result, following removal of the undeveloped silver halide crystals by the fixer, is a deposition of metallic silver on the film itself corresponding to the initial photon interactions.

The greater the deposition of metallic silver, the less transmission of light through the film. As the transmission of light through an object decreases, we say that the object is increasing in density. Density itself can be defined as the amount of darkening on a film expressed mathematically as the logarithm base ten of the intensity of the incident light divided by the intensity of the light after passing through the film, or

$$D = \log \frac{I_o}{I}$$

where I_o = incident light intensity
I = light intensity transmitted through the object

Problem If the light intensity is decreased to 10 percent of its initial intensity as it passes through a film, what is the density of the film?

Answer Assume that the light intensity is 100 percent (I_o) when there is no film.

$$D = \log \frac{I_o}{I}$$

$$D = \log \frac{100\%}{10\%} = \log 10$$

The log of 10 equals 1. Therefore

$$D = 1$$

Problem What would be the density if 1 percent of the light was transmitted through the film?

Answer

$$D = \log \frac{I_o}{I}$$

$$D = \log \frac{100}{1} = \log 100$$

The log of 100 equals 2. Therefore

$$D = 2$$

Note that every increase in density by one unit is caused by a decrease of light transmission by a factor of 10.

Usually the densities used in diagnostic radiology vary from 0.4 to more than 3.0.

Radiographic Contrast

Radiographic contrast can, for the purposes of this discussion, be defined as the density difference between the two points of interest, or

$$\text{Contrast } (C) = D_2 - D_1$$

The greater the density difference, the greater will be the radiographic contrast.

Characteristic Curve

A curve describing the density of film as a function of the exposure is known as a characteristic curve. It is also sometimes referred to as an H and D curve (named after Hurter and Driffield) or as a D-log E curve (dose–log exposure curve). Figure 7-1 illustrates a typical characteristic curve.

The actual position of the curve on the chart for each film is not a

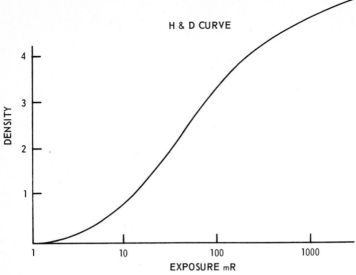

Figure 7-1 Typical characteristic curve.

constant, but varies as a function of kilovolts peak; i.e., the curve will shift to the left as kVp is decreased and move to the right as kVp is increased.

SPECIFIC FACTORS AFFECTING RADIOGRAPHIC IMAGES

Table 7-1 lists factors which affect radiographic images. Please note that while both radiographic contrast and definition each affect the radiographic image, they are mutually independent of each other.

The greater the radiographic contrast, the greater the radiographic detail. The greater the definition (sharpness), the greater the radiographic detail.

Radiographic Contrast

Radiographic contrast has been previously defined as the difference of densities between the two points of interest, or

$$C = D_2 - D_1$$

Radiographic contrast itself is determined by both subject contrast and film contrast. As subject contrast or film contrast increases, radiographic contrast also increases.

Table 7-1 Factors Affecting Radiographic Images

Radiographic Contrast		Definition (Sharpness)	
Subject contrast	Film contrast	Geometric Factors	Radiographic mottle
1. Subject	1. Film itself	1. Focal spot size	1. Graininess
2. kVp (radiation quality)	2. Development procedure	2. Source-to-image-receptor distance	2. Quantum mottle
3. Scattered radiation	3. Exposure	3. Subject-to-image-receptor distance	
		4. Film-screen contact	
		5. Screen speed	
		6. Motion	

Subject Contrast Subject contrast can be defined as the differences in absorption of the radiation by the part under examination. Subject contrast is affected by three factors.

The Subject Itself In order for there to be any subject contrast, the subject itself must be either of different thicknesses, atomic numbers, or densities. If not, as in the example of a thin uniform piece of plastic, it would appear on a radiograph to be without any contrast.

kVp (Quality) The greater the quality of the beam, the less is the subject contrast (and therefore the radiographic contrast). Figure 7-2 demonstrates the effect of changing kilovoltage on subject contrast.

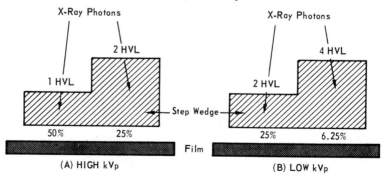

Figure 7-2 Effect of changing kilovoltage on subject contrast.

Let us assume that in situation A the subject is being x-rayed at a high kVp using a highly filtered beam. The thicker part of the step wedge represents a dense or thick part of the subject, while the thinner portion represents a less dense or thinner part of the subject. We will also make the further assumption that the thicker part represents two half-value layers (HVLs),* while the thinner part represents 1 HVL. Therefore, 50 percent (1 HVL) of the beam will be transmitted through the thinner part while 25 percent (2 HVLs) will penetrate the thicker part. This is a *difference of 2 to 1 in terms of exposure to the respective parts of the film.* If, as in example B, the kVp were decreased (lower-quality beam), the penetrating capability of the beam would also decrease. We can assume that as the penetrating capability decreases, the same object will act as if it were a greater number of HVLs. Let us assume that by decreasing the kVp, we now have 2 HVLs in the thinner part and 4 HVLs in the thicker part. Therefore, as illustrated in Fig. 7-2, the intensity of the thinner part would be 25 percent of the initial exposure rate (2 HVLs), while that under the thicker portion would be 6.25 percent of the initial exposure rate (4 HVLs). Thus, in this case of the lower beam quality, using the same object, there is a 4:1 *difference* (25/6.25) in terms of exposure to the respective parts of the film. The latter situation (a 4:1 difference of exposures to the film) results in a *greater* density difference (contrast) to the film. Therefore, as illustrated in Fig. 7-2, as kVp decreases, subject contrast increases; conversely, as kVp increases, subject contrast decreases.

Scattered Radiation   Scattered radiation can add a uniform exposure to the film but does not add a uniform density. This results in decreased contrast, as explained in Fig. 7-3.

In this hypothetical example, the entrance exposure is 100 mR, while with minimum scatter the film under the bone and tissue are exposed to 2 and 5 mR respectively. Using the characteristic curve (Fig. 7-4) for the film, note that the areas of the film have a density of approximately 1.6 and 2.4, or a contrast of 0.8 as represented by the density differences.

If, for example, by improper collimation the film is additionally exposed to 4 mR of scattered radiation (an arbitrary figure), then the two film areas would have, as illustrated in Fig. 7-5, 6 and 9 mR, respectively.

Note in Fig. 7-6 that the characteristic curve indicates that the densities under the film are approximately 2.5 and 3.1, respectively, or a contrast of about 0.6 as represented by the density difference.

---

* HVL—half-value layer, or that quantity of shielding or filtration required to decrease the quantity of radiation by one-half.

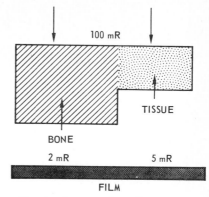

Figure 7-3 Minimum scatter on film due to properly collimated beam.

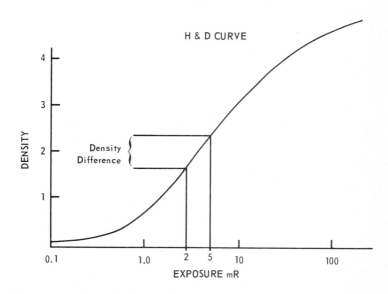

Figure 7-4 Density difference with minimum scatter.

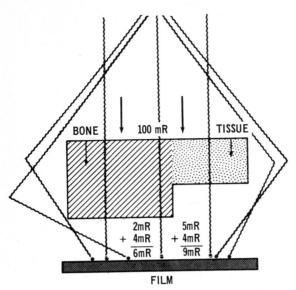

Figure 7-5 Scatter due to improperly collimated beam.

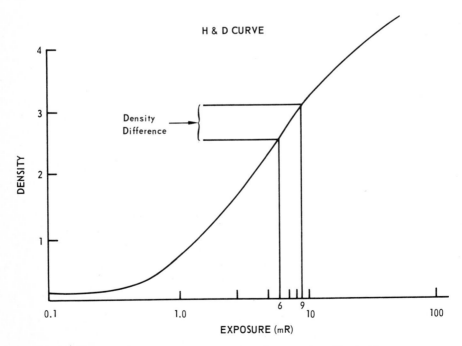

Figure 7-6 Density difference with scatter from improperly collimated beam.

As illustrated in Fig. 7-6, increased scattered radiation decreases subject contrast, thereby also decreasing radiographic contrast which causes decreased radiographic image detail. This effect can be minimized by the use of proper collimation. Grids also improve image quality by removing scattered photons which would decrease subject contrast.

Film Contrast   Film contrast is the contrast developed which is characteristic of both the film and the processing. It is affected by three factors.

The Film Itself   In the example of the step wedge illustrated above as Fig. 7-3, 2 and 5 mR are received respectively by the film. In Fig. 7-7, the characteristic curves of two different manufacturers' films illustrate the different contrasts developed.

Note that for the same exposure to the films, type A has a greater contrast (density difference) than type B.

Development Procedure   The film contrast can be affected by processing time. For example, if the proper time-temperature recommendations of the manufacturer are not followed, the maximum film contrast is not

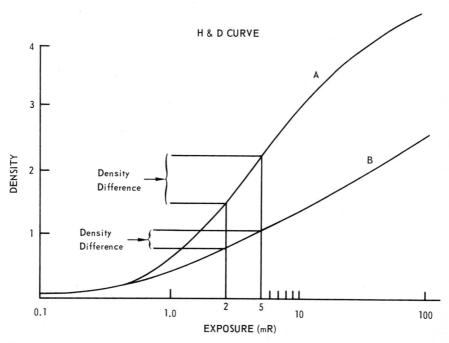

Figure 7-7 Effect of film type on contrast.

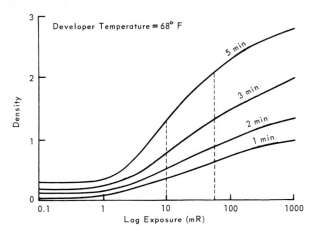

Figure 7-8 Effect of development time on contrast. (Bureau of Radiological Health, Food and Drug Administration, U.S. Department of Health, Education and Welfare.)

achieved. This concept is illustrated in Fig. 7-8. If we arbitrarily use approximately 10 and 60 mR as our reference points, note that it takes a full 5 min for the maximum contrast or density difference to be fully developed.

Exposure   If, by not using 2- and 5-mR exposures as our reference points, the film is underexposed, i.e., using 0.2 and 0.5 mR, respectively, then not only will the density be decreased but also the contrast, as illustrated in Fig. 7-9.

Definition (Sharpness)

Definition (sharpness) can be defined as the abruptness of transition in film density. Definition is influenced by both geometric factors and radiographic mottle.

Geometric factors

Focal Spot Size   As the focal spot decreases in size, the sharpness of the image increases. Conversely, with the use of a large focal spot, the sharpness of the image decreases. This is explained in Fig. 7-10.

The large penumbra, or vague borderline area around the umbra under the large focal spot, is due to x-rays striking the outer edges from all regions of the focal area.

Source-to-Image-Receptor Distance   As the source-to-image-receptor distance (SID) increases, the x-ray beam becomes more parallel. Conversely,

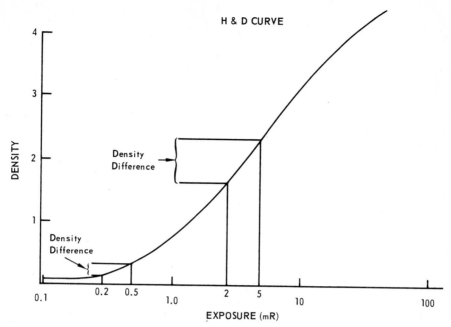

Figure 7-9 Effect of exposure on contrast.

as the SID decreases, the beam becomes more divergent. The parallel beam (greater SID) will record an image that is sharper and with less distortion.

Subject-to-Image-Receptor Distance   As the subject-to-image-receptor distance decreases, the resulting radiographic is both sharper and more representative in size of the object being radiographed.

Film-Screen Contact   The closer the contact between the film and the screen, the sharper the recorded image of the film.

As illustrated in Fig. 7-11, the closer the screen-film contact, the less the overlapping coning of light. Overlapping of light will result in a less sharp image since the density within the area has been contributed to by light from two separate screen interactions.

Screen Speed   In general, the thicker the screen, the faster its speed. The speed of the screen is also influenced, but to a lesser extent, by the crystal size itself. Figure 7-12 illustrates how screen thickness influences both the speed of the screen and the sharpness of the recorded image.

The high-speed screen is thicker than the slow-speed screen. This means that there is a greater probability of interaction with the high-speed screen.

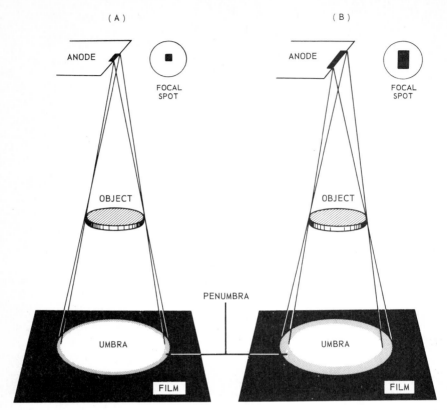

Figure 7-10 Effect of focal spot size on sharpness. (Bureau of Radiological Health, Food and Drug Administration, U.S. Department of Health, Education and Welfare.)

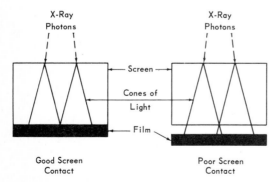

Figure 7-11 Effect of screen-film contact on sharpness. (Bureau of Radiological Health, Food and Drug Administration, U.S. Department of Health, Education and Welfare.)

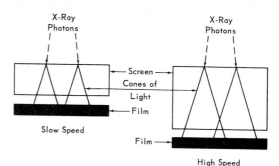

Figure 7-12 Effect of screen speed on sharpness. (Bureau of Radiological Health, Food and Drug Administration, U.S. Department of Health, Education and Welfare.)

The greater the probability of interaction, the greater the number of light flashes reaching the film and therefore the greater the apparent speed of the screen.

However, as the speed of the screen increases, there is some loss of sharpness of the fluorescent image. In the above example of the slow-speed screen we have two hypothetical interactions occurring near the outside surface. From these two interactions, two flashes of light are generated which produce two distinct areas of blackening when they reach the film.

In the example of the high-speed screen, let the two same hypothetical interactions occur near the surface of the screen. Again two flashes of light are generated which, because they have a further distance to travel prior to reaching the film, will cone out such that they can actually overlap each other on the film. This means that part of the darkening on the film is contributed to by two different initial interactions in the screen, resulting in an image which is reduced in sharpness.

Motion Motion can cause blurring. Therefore, the time of exposure should be as short as possible in order to "freeze" any movement.

Radiographic Mottle

Graininess The actual grains of silver halide in a film emulsion are approximately 1 micrometer in size. This means that they are far too small to be seen by the unaided eye. What we call graininess is actually the chance accumulation of developed grains.

As the kVp (quality) of the beam is increased, the average energy of the x-ray photons is also increased. This increased energy is passed on to the photoelectrons (or Compton electrons) which are liberated by the interaction of the photon with the film. Because the photoelectron has greater energy, it can interact with more crystals to form additional latent images. If the crystals, by chance, are in close proximity to each other, when they are developed they will appear to be one visible dark area on the film which can look like a dot.

Therefore, as the kVp increases, graininess may also increase with a resultant loss in sharpness.

Quantum Mottle   Quantum mottle is actually a rather recent development in terms of becoming apparent on images.

X-rays do not leave the tube as waves—like sound waves or waves on an ocean. Instead, they are actually small discrete bundles of energy called quanta or photons. Each photon has its own energy and associated wavelength.

As faster films (or electronic recording devices) were developed, the number of photons required to form an image was reduced.

Since the quantity of photons produced per unit area is not evenly distributed but is a statistical function, at any point in time one minute area of film may receive a greater quantity of photons than a different adjacent area.

When slower image-recording devices were used, this did not make too much of a difference since the large number of photons required tended to dampen or smooth out any major percent statistical variations. However, with the newer high-speed image-recording systems, it is possible to actually see the quantum mottle effect caused by the "relatively small" number of photons reaching the film and therefore the larger percent variation of adjacent areas in terms of photons received.

This becomes visible as small areas of quantum mottle or a type of pattern on the film itself with the net result of a decrease in sharpness. A slower image-recording system will have less quantum mottle, therefore greater sharpness, but at the price of increased radiation exposure.

When screens are used, there is also a contributing factor of screen mottle itself. Screen mottle is caused by the inherent random distribution of crystals within the screen.

QUESTIONS

7-1   If 0.1 percent of the incident light is transmitted through a film, what is the film's density?

7-2   What is the approximate range of densities used in diagnostic radiology?

7-3 If, upon development, a radiograph is too dark (overexposed), should you retake it using the same machine settings but developing it for a shorter period of time? Why? What effect would this shortened development time have on the contrast?

7-4 What happens to the contrast of the radiograph (gray scale) as you increase kVp (quality)? Why?

7-5 Explain why scattered radiation does *not* add uniform density to a radiograph.

7-6 Will the use of a grid increase or decrease the image detail? Why?

7-7 Would you expect a greater quantum mottle effect from a high-speed screen–film combination or from a non-screen film?

7-8 Explain why we still need different possible film-screen combinations even though image detail of the combinations can vary appreciably.

7-9 What is meant by graininess? How is it affected by kVp? Why?

7-10 Make a list of the factors under your control as a radiologic technologist that affect image detail.

REFERENCES

1 Moe, H.J., et al.: "Radiation Safety Technician Training Course Manual," ANL-7291 Rev. 1, National Technical Information Service, U.S. Department of Commerce, 1972.

2 Kodak: "The Fundamentals of Radiography," 11th ed., Eastman Kodak Company, Rochester, N.Y., 1968.

3 Frankel, R.: "Factors Affecting Radiographic Image," PHS training fascicle TP-467, 1968.

4 Oman, R.: "An Introduction to Radiologic Science," McGraw-Hill, New York, 1975.

5 Kodak: "Sensitometric Properties of X-Ray Films," Eastman Kodak Company, Rochester, N.Y., M1-2.

6 Lecture notes of a presentation by George M. Corney, Radiological Markets Division, Eastman Kodak Company.

Chapter 8

Basic Principles of Radiation Protection

Objectives

The student learns the basic fundamental concepts of radiation protection. The student should

    1 Know about the general protection methods from external sources of ionizing radiation
    2 Be aware of the general protection methods from internal sources of ionizing radiation

    There are two potential sources of radiation exposure to patients and operators: (1) external and (2) internal.

EXTERNAL SOURCES

By this terminology it is meant that the source of the radiation is located outside the body, e.g., x-ray machines and cobalt-60 teletherapy units.

No matter how sophisticated one becomes in radiation protection, there are basically only three ways to protect either patients or operators from excessive radiation exposure from external sources. They are *time, distance,* and *shielding.*

Time

Radiation exposure is directly related to time. For example, if the exposure rate is 25 mR/h, an exposure of 25 mR will be received if the individual remains for 1 h. Therefore, for purposes of radiation protection, it is prudent to minimize the total time of exposure.

There are circumstances where time will be one of the most important protection factors available. For example, in the loading of radium nasopharyngeal applicators or the insertion of radioactive sources in the body, it is absolutely essential that the procedures be as efficient as possible in order to minimize the time of exposure. This is illustrated by the following problem.

Problem If the exposure rate to the technologist is 50 mR/h while loading a radium nasopharyngeal applicator, what will be his exposure if the procedure takes 10 min? Suppose, through practice (dry runs), he was able to reduce the time to 7 min, what would be the reduction of exposure?

Answer

$$\frac{50 \text{ mR}}{h} \times \frac{1 \text{ h}}{60 \text{ min}} \times 10 \text{ min} = 8.3 \text{ mR}$$

If the time is reduced to 7 min, then

$$\frac{50 \text{ mR}}{h} \times \frac{1 \text{ h}}{60 \text{ min}} \times 7 \text{ min} = 5.8 \text{ mR}$$

The mR reduction would be

$$8.3 \text{ mR} - 5.8 \text{ mR} = 2.5 \text{ mR}$$

Distance

Intuitively, we know that the farther away we are from a source of radiation, the less exposure we receive. Specifically, the intensity of radiation varies inversely as the square of the distance; i.e., if the distance from the source is

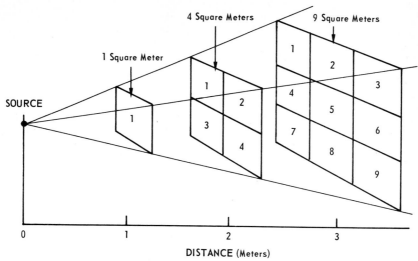

Figure 8-1 Inverse-square law.

doubled, the intensity of the radiation will be decreased by a factor of 4. Figure 8-1 will explain why.

Note in this three-dimensional sketch that the solid angle subtended by the source has all the radiation going through 1 m² at 1 m from the source. As we increase the distance to 2 m, since the beam is divergent all of the radiation that was going through 1 m² (radiation flux) is now going through 4 m². Therefore, the intensity per *each* square meter has been decreased by a factor of 4.

Using the same line of reasoning, we note that at 3 m from the source the amount of radiation that was going through 1 m² (at 1 m from the source) is now going through 9 m². Therefore the intensity per *each* square meter has been decreased by a factor of 9.

Again, note that the intensity of radiation varies inversely as the square of the distance from the source. In the examples noted above, as we doubled the distance, we decreased the exposure by a factor of 4, 2^2; as we tripled the distance, we decreased the exposure by a factor of 9, 3^2.

Since the amount of exposure received varies *inversely* as the *square* of the distance, small changes in distance can result in relatively large changes in exposures. The actual exposures at various distances can be calculated by the use of the following formula:

$$\frac{X_1}{X_2} = \frac{d_2^2}{d_1^2}$$

where X_1 = exposure rate at a point d_1
   d_1 = distance of X_1 from the source of the radiation
   X_2 = exposure rate at a point d_2
   d_2 = distance of X_2 from the source of the radiation

Problem   If the exposure rate at 50 cm from the x-ray machine is 50 R/h, what will be the exposure rate at 250 cm from the x-ray machine?

Answer   Substituting in the formula for the inverse-square law,

X_1 = 50 R/h
d_1 = 50 cm
X_2 = unknown
d_2 = 250 cm

$$\frac{X_1}{X_2} = \frac{d_2^2}{d_1^2}$$

$$\frac{50 \text{ R/h}}{X_2} = \frac{(250)^2}{(50)^2}$$

$$\frac{50}{X_2} = \frac{62,000}{2,500}$$

We then cross-multiply to obtain

$$62,500 X_2 = 125,000$$
$$X_2 = 2\text{R/h}$$

Shielding

Intuitively, we realize that the thicker the shield, the greater the protection. We also recall that for the most part, x-ray photons in the diagnostic energy range interact with matter mostly by the photoelectric effect and, to a lesser extent, by Compton scatter.

Since the probability of interaction by the photoelectric effect varies approximately (in the diagnostic range) as Z^3 of the absorber (Z number equals the atomic number), the greater the atomic number, the greater the probability of the photoelectric effect occurring. For example, lead (atomic number = 82) is much more efficient in removing photons from a beam than aluminum (atomic number = 13). Since the probability of the photoelectric effect in the diagnostic x-ray range varies approximately as Z^3, we can compare their efficiency as a shield by comparing their respective atomic numbers: lead, $Z = 82$; aluminum, $Z = 13$, or

$$Z^3 = \left(\frac{82}{13}\right)^3 = (6.31)^3 = 250$$

Therefore, the same mass of lead will be about 250 times more efficient in removing the low-energy photons found in diagnostic x-rays by the photo-electric effect than aluminum. This is why lead or other high Z number material, rather than aluminum, is used as shielding in diagnostic x-ray suites.

Half-Value Layer (HVL) A concept that is very important for radio-logic technologists to understand is that of half-value layer (HVL). The HVL can be defined as that quantity of shielding (or filtration) which will decrease the original intensity of the beam by one-half. For example, Fig. 8-2 shows that without any shielding, the exposure rate at 2 m from the radioactive source is 20 R/h.

Keeping all other factors constant, if we place absorbers midway between the source and the detection instrument, there is a decrease in the instrument reading. When the reading has decreased (because of the addition of the absorbers) to one-half of its original intensity, as illustrated in Fig. 8-3 (in the example cited above, from 20 R/h to 10 R/h), we measure the thickness of the added absorbers. This thickness is known as the half-value layer. Therefore, one half-value layer of an absorber will decrease the intensity by 50 percent.

Problem The half-value layer (HVL) for cobalt-60 in terms of lead is 1.2 cm. If the initial exposure rate at a point outside of a teletherapy room is 8 mR/h, what will be the exposure rate, if two half-value layers of lead (i.e., 1.2 cm $\times$ 2 = 2.4 cm) are added to the walls of the teletherapy room?

Answer Since *each* half-value layer decreases the exposure rate by one-half (50 percent), one HVL (1.2 cm) will decrease the exposure rate from 8 mR/h to 4 mR/h. However, we now add a second HVL of lead so that the 4 mR/h is decreased again by one-half (50 percent) to become 2 mR/h. Therefore, two HVLs of lead in the example cited above will decrease the exposure rate to 2 mR/h.

Remember, each added half-value layer of absorber will decrease the exposure rate by one-half of what it was before the addition of the half-value layer.

Problem How many HVLs of an absorber are required to reduce the exposure rate to less than 1 percent (0.01) of its initial intensity?

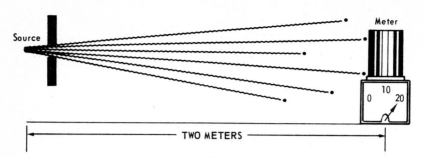

Figure 8-2 Exposure with no added absorbers.

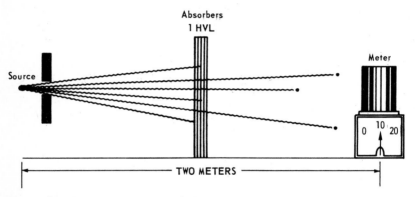

Figure 8-3 Exposure with 1 HVL of added absorbers.

Answer

HVL	Intensity, %
0	100
1	50
2	25
3	12.5
4	6.25
5	3.125
6	1.56
7	0.78

Therefore, 7 half-value layers are required to decrease the exposure rate to less than 1 percent (0.01) of its initial intensity. Since the HVL for *radio-isotopes* is a *constant*, in order to obtain a decrease of exposure rate to less than 1 percent of its initial intensity (or stating it in a different manner, a protection factor of 100 times), 7 HVLs of lead are required. If 1 HVL of lead in terms of radium-226 is 1.66 cm, then 7 HVLs would be 1.66 cm × 7 = 11.62 cm; 11.62 cm (4.57 in) is slightly larger than the width of a brick.

Although the HVL concept for shielding calculations is beyond the immediate scope of this text, suffice it to say that the health physicist can calculate shielding requirements for teletherapy suites or other radioisotopes based on the respective HVLs of the shield in respect to the isotope. For further information on the subject of isotope shielding, the reader is encouraged to review the references listed at the end of this chapter.

As stated above, the HVL for radioisotopes is a constant. This is *not* the case for diagnostic x-rays, For x-rays, the HVL increases as additional absorbers are added.

As the reader recalls, x-ray photons (by the nature of their bremsstrahlung production) are not all of the same energy. In fact, a spectrum of energies is produced.

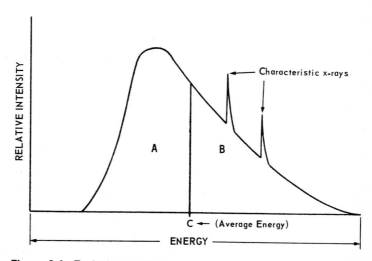

Figure 8-4 Typical x-ray spectrum.

TYPICAL X-RAY SPECTRUM

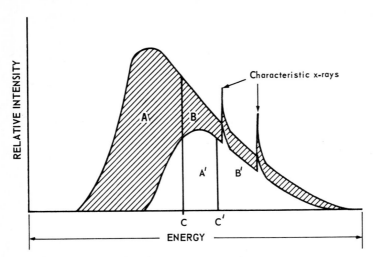

Figure 8-5 Effect of absorbers on x-ray spectrum.

If we divide the spectrum into two equal parts, A and B, then the *average* energy could be described as point C. Therefore initially the x-ray beam appears to have a HVL of a monoenergetic beam of photons of energy C.

However, as soon as absorbers are added, the average energy increases (because of the interaction of x-rays with matter).

As absorbers are added, the lower-energy photons (in part A) are mostly completely absorbed by the photoelectric effect, while the higher-energy photons* (in part B) have a greater probability of interaction by Compton scattering or of passing through the absorbers with no interaction at all. The net result is that the lower-energy photons are preferentially removed from the beam, resulting in a spectrum now described by A^1 and B^1 with a new average energy of C^1. Since C^1 is a greater *average* energy than C^1, the beam is now acting as if it were of a higher monoenergetic energy. Since *the greater the photon energy, the more absorbers it would take to decrease the intensity by one-half (HVL),* as we add additional absorbers to an x-ray beam:

---

* It is suggested that the modern scientific notation of high- or low-energy photons be used to replace the older terminology of hard or soft x-rays.

1   The average energy increases.
2   The HVL increases.
3   The intensity decreases since part of the beam is removed by the added absorbers.

Because of the increasing HVL of x-rays as a function of added absorbers, the health physicist cannot use exponential equations to calculate primary diagnostic x-ray shielding requirements. Instead, barrier requirements are computed using a series of x-ray transmission curves for lead or concrete. In order to calculate the necessary shielding, the following information is required:

1   Is the area to be shielded a controlled area? A controlled area is "a defined area in which the exposure of persons to radiation is under the supervision of a Radiation Protection Supervisor. (This implies that a controlled area is one that requires control of access, occupancy and working conditions for radiation protection purposes.)"
2   Is the unit in question used for therapy or diagnosis? If for diagnosis, is it a radiographic or fluoroscopic unit?
3   What is the maximum kVp of the unit?
4   What is the workload of the unit?
5   Is the area to be shielded from the primary beam or from secondary radiation (scatter and leakage)?
6   What is the distance from the unit (and scatterer in the case of secondary radiation protection barriers) to the area to be protected?
7   What is the use factor? The use factor is the "fraction of the workload during which the radiation under consideration is directed at a particular barrier."
8   What is the occupancy factor? The occupancy factor is "the factor by which the workload should be multiplied to correct for the degree of occupancy of the area in question while the source is 'ON'."*
9   What is the composition of the planned or the existing walls?

Using the appropriate above information the health physicist can calculate the necessary shielding requirements. Although the actual computations are beyond the immediate scope of this text, interested readers are encouraged to review the references listed at the end of this chapter with special attention to be given to NCRP Report 34.

* NCRP, Medical X-ray and Gamma-Ray Protection for Energies up to 10 Mev, *NCRP Report* 34, pp. 43, 44, and 46, 1970.

INTERNAL SOURCES

Although the basic radiation protection aspects of this text are intended to be healing arts x-ray, the following brief discussion is provided in order to acquaint the reader with internal sources.*

Internal sources are those in which the source of the radiation is located inside the body; e.g., iodine-131 incorporated in the thyroid gland.

Radionuclide Uptake

It is prudent that procedures be utilized by the technologist in order to minimize the inadvertent uptake of radionuclides by the body.

The following are routes of possible body uptake of radionuclides: ingestion, inhalation, absorption.

Ingestion   Radioactive material could be inadvertently ingested from contaminated hands, food, or utensils. It is absolutely essential that personnel thoroughly wash their hands prior to eating, smoking, or leaving work. In addition, eating, smoking, and storage or the preparation of food in a laboratory which contains unsealed sources are prohibited.

To avoid the accidental ingestion of radionuclides, routine pipetting by mouth should not be permitted.

Inhalation   Radioactive material which has been inhaled may not only be exhaled (therefore no body uptake) but also be deposited in the lungs and (for most nuclides) eventually either absorbed systemically or swallowed.

To avoid the inhalation of radioactive materials, smoking is absolutely prohibited in laboratories which contain unsealed sources. Cigarettes, for example, could be placed on a contaminated workbench which could result in the inadvertent uptake by inhalation (or ingestion) of an isotope.

In addition, the proper use of a radiological hood along with air monitoring systems will minimize air contamination. It is suggested that the technologist utilize the services of the institute *radiation safety officer* (RSO) not only for questions pertaining to the hood and air monitoring systems, but for all matters concerning radiation safety.

Absorption   Certain radionuclides (e.g., tritium), depending upon their chemical form, can also be absorbed directly through the skin. To minimize the possibility of absorption (and skin contamination), protective gloves should be worn whenever there is a possibility of hand contamination.

---

* For additional information, the reader is especially encouraged to review the publication: Williams, K. D., et al., "Reduction of Radiation Exposure in Nuclear Medicine," Public Health Service Publication 999-RH-30, 1967.

Good Housekeeping In order to be as efficient as possible and to minimize any radiation dose, the technologist should practice cleanliness and neatness. He should also practice the procedures involved by "dry runs." In addition the work area should, following the advice of the radiation safety officer, be prepared to handle any accidental spills. This may include working in stainless steel trays lined with heavy absorbent paper and/or absorbent paper strategically placed throughout specified work areas. There should also be proper survey and laboratory instrumentation available in order to monitor for contamination. The type of instrumentation needed depends upon the isotopes used. For example, alpha detectors should be available to monitor any possible contamination from alpha emitters. A beta-gamma survey instrument such as a Geiger counter is sufficient for most of the other commonly used isotopes. However special monitoring techniques are needed for low-energy beta emitters such as tritium.

Emergency Procedures Each facility should have a plan which deals with emergency situations such as radioactive liquid spills or the loss of powdered or gaseous radioactive material. The technologist is urged to become familiar with the plan and to consult the RSO of the facility on any questions concerning its implementation.

QUESTIONS

8-1 Of the three basic methods of protection from external sources of ionizing radiation, which do you consider to be the most important? Why?

8-2 If the average maximum permissible dose equivalent is 100 mrems per week, how long can an occupationally exposed individual remain in an area if the exposure rate is 15 mR/h?

8-3 Explain why the half-value layer for diagnostic x-rays increases as filtration is added.

8-4 If a wood wall is 1 cm thick, will an additional 1 cm of wood (so now the wall is twice as thick or 2 cm) decrease the exposure rate through it by a factor of 2?

8-5 If the exposure rate at a point 22 cm from a source is 250 mR/h, what will be the exposure rate at a point 10 cm from the source?

8-6 Draw the approximate x-ray spectrum you would expect of a beam that has penetrated through a lead tube housing.

8-7 What should one of your first responses be in the event of a liquid spill in a radioisotope laboratory?

8-8 If the half-value layer (HVL) for lead in terms of radium is 1.66 cm, how much lead (thickness) is required to decrease the gamma radiation to 12.5 percent of the initial intensity?

8-9 Name three possible methods for the accidental uptake of radionuclides. Discuss protection methods to minimize each of these possibilities.

8-10 Should lead aprons (0.5 mm of lead equivalent) be utilized for personal protection when working with radium? Why?

REFERENCES

1 Oman, Robert M.: "An Introduction to Radiologic Science," McGraw-Hill, New York, 1975.

2 Moe, H. J., et al.: "Radiation Safety Technician Training Course Manual," ANL-7291, Rev. 1, National Technical Information Service, U.S. Department of Commerce, 1972.

3 Cember, H.: "Introduction to Health Physics," Pergamon, New York, 1969.

4 NCRP: Medical X-Ray and Gamma-Ray Protection for Energies up to 10 MeV, *NCRP Report* 34, NCRP Publications, 1970.

5 NCRP: Protection against Radiation from Brachytherapy Sources, *NCRP Report* 40, NCRP Publications, 1972.

6 Blatz, H.: "Radiation Hygiene Handbook," McGraw-Hill, New York, 1959.

7 Andrews, H.: "Radiation Biophysics," Prentice-Hall, Englewood Cliffs, N.J., 1962.

8 Williams, K. D., et al,: "Reduction of Radiation Exposure in Nuclear Medicine," Public Health Service Publication 999-RH-30, 1967.

9 Granlund, R. W.: "The Changing Responsibilities of the Radiation Safety Officer," presented at the 1973 meeting of the Health Physics Society.

10 "Environmental Aspects of the Hospital," vol. III, "Safety Fundamentals," Public Health Service Publication 930-C-17, 1967.

11 "Inhalation Risks from Radioactive Contaminants," chapter 7, International Atomic Energy Agency, Vienna, 1973.

Chapter 9

Methods to Minimize Diagnostic X-Ray Exposure to Patients and Operators

Objectives

The student learns the basic methods of minimizing diagnostic x-ray exposure to patients and operators. The student should

1 Know six specific radiographic techniques that can minimize patient exposure

2 Understand the correlation of the above six techniques with operator exposure

3 Be able to describe additional methods to minimize radiographic operator exposure

4 Know the radiation protection requirements while using mobile radiographic equipment

5 Be aware of fluoroscopic operator precautions

The previous chapter discussed the general principles of radiation protection. This chapter will cover specific methods to minimize excessive radiation exposure to both patients and operators from diagnostic radiology.

RADIOGRAPHIC UNITS

Methods to Minimize Patient Exposure

In addition to techniques such as proper positioning and proper patient instruction, there are several specific ways to further minimize patient exposure.

Proper Collimation The maximum allowable dimensions of the x-ray beam should be approximately the size of the image receptor. The amount of variance permitted from the actual image-receptor size depends upon the specific state or federal regulations for the equipment.

Even though state or federal regulations have a maximum allowable x-ray beam size as a function of image-receptor size, the x-ray operator can further minimize patient exposure by limiting the x-ray beam to the area of clinical interest.

With the use of optimum collimation practices, only tissues of the body in which there is a diagnostic interest will be in the primary beam. This is very important since there can be hundreds of times more exposure to tissues in the primary beam as compared to that received as scattered x-rays by adjacent tissues.

A secondary benefit from properly collimated x-ray beams is less scattering of x-rays reaching the film. This results in greater subject contrast and in a higher-quality radiograph (see Chap. 7).

The federal x-ray standard requires that general-purpose fixed radiographic units manufactured after August 1, 1974 have positive beam-limiting devices which will either cause automatic adjustment of the field to the image-receptor size within a certain time period or prevent production of x-rays until adjustment is completed.

Units manufactured prior to August 1, 1974 must meet the individual state collimation requirements. Some states require variable rectangular collimators with a beam-defining light, while others may permit a circular cone to be used. The reader should contact his respective state radiation control program for any questions pertaining to specific requirements.

The following problem illustrates how a manufacturer can calculate the dimensions of a lead diaphragm to be used with a specific film size and a fixed source-to-image-receptor distance (SID).

Problem If the SID for a cystographic unit is fixed at 40 in, what size lead diaphragm, to be used as a collimator, should be inserted to limit the beam size to 14 $\times$ 17 in?

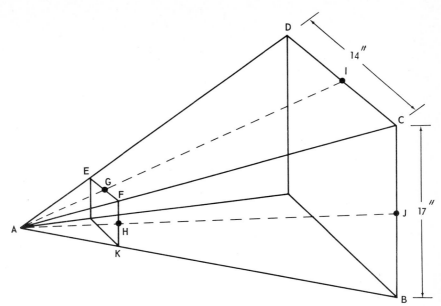

Figure 9-1 Similar triangles method to calculate dimensions of a diaphragm.

Answer The manufacturer measures the distance from the tube target to where the collimator (lead diaphragm) is to be placed. With this information, using the geometry theorem that similar parts of similar triangles are similar, the exact size of the collimator can be calculated. This is illustrated in Fig. 9-1.

If through measurements it is determined that the lead diaphragm is to be placed 4 in from the target *(A)*, then $\overline{AG}$ = 4 in and $\overline{AH}$ = 4 in.

The 14 × 17 in film is 40 in from the target. This means that $\overline{AI}$ = 40 in and that $\overline{AJ}$ = 40 in.

To calculate the actual dimensions of the lead diaphragm first determine one side and then the other.

The first side will be the length that determines the 17-in dimension of the film, or $\overline{CB}$. This corresponds to $\overline{FK}$ in the lead diaphragm. The triangle *ABC* is similar to the triangle *AKF*. Therefore, similar parts of similar triangles are similar; i.e., $\overline{FK}$ is similar to $\overline{CB}$ and $\overline{AH}$ is similar to $\overline{AJ}$. Since similar parts of the similar triangles are similar, the following proportion is established:

$$\frac{\overline{FK}}{\overline{CB}} = \frac{\overline{AH}}{\overline{AJ}}$$

We know that $\overline{AH}$ = 4 in, $\overline{AJ}$ = 40 in, and that $\overline{CB}$ = 17 in. The only unknown is $\overline{FK}$.

$$\frac{X}{17} = \frac{4}{40}$$
$$40x = 68$$
$$x = 1.7 \text{ in}$$

Therefore one side of the lead diaphragm should be cut such that it is 1.7 in in length.

The other length of the film is 14 in, or $\overline{DC}$. This corresponds to $\overline{EF}$ in the lead diaphragm. Using the two similar triangles ADC and AEF, we can set up a proportion of the similar parts; i.e., $\overline{AG}$ is similar to $\overline{AI}$, while $\overline{EF}$ is similar to $\overline{DC}$, or

$$\frac{\overline{EF}}{\overline{DC}} = \frac{\overline{AG}}{\overline{AI}}$$

We know that $\overline{AG}$ = 4 in, $\overline{AI}$ = 40 in, and that $\overline{DC}$ = 14 in. The only unknown is $\overline{EF}$.

$$\frac{X}{14} = \frac{4}{40}$$
$$40x = 56$$
$$x = 1.4 \text{ in}$$

Therefore, if a lead diaphragm is constructed by the manufacturer such that it is 1.4 × 1.7 in and placed 4 in from the target, the resulting x-ray beam, 40 in from the target, will be 14 × 17 in.

Gonad Shields   The purpose of a gonad shield is to minimize radiation dose to the reproductive organs when they are in or near (within about 5 cm) a properly collimated beam. The primary beam dose reduction can vary from 90 percent with the use of shaped contact shields on male patients to a 50 percent reduction by the use of flat contact shielding on female patients. A radiograph with a gonad shield in position is illustrated in Fig. 9–2.

At the present time the clinical procedures for the appropriate use of testicular shields has been better demonstrated than for ovarian shielding.

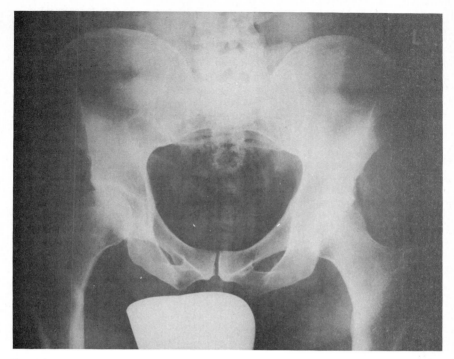

Figure 9-2 Radiograph showing gonad shielding. (Bureau of Radiological Health, Food and Drug Administration, U.S. Department of Health, Education and Welfare.)

However, some individuals have been successfully utilizing ovarian shielding for selected views in some examinations.

Types of Gonad Shields There are currently available three generic types of gonad shields: flat contact shields, shadow shields, and shaped contact shields.

Flat contact shields. This shield can be constructed from a lead-impregnated material. It can be directly placed on or can be taped over the gonads. The flat contact shield is most effective when it is used for posterior/anterior (PA) or anterior/posterior (AP) views. Because the flat contact shielding is difficult to maintain in place, it is not recommended for fluoroscopy or for nonrecumbent projections.

Shadow shields. A shadow shield (see Fig. 9-3) is suspended in the light field of the beam-defining light over the area of a patient to be radiographed and is composed of a radiopaque material. A shadow of the shield is cast by the beam-defining light. If the beam-defining light is accurately

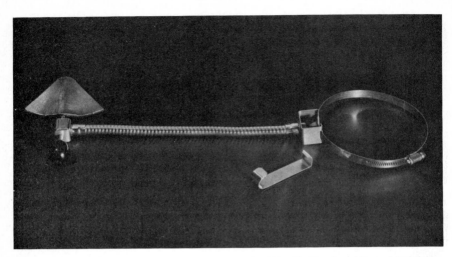

Figure 9-3 Shadow shield. (Bureau of Radiological Health, Food and Drug Administration, U.S. Department of Health, Education and Welfare.)

aligned, the area of the body under the shadow will be protected from the primary x-ray beam. The shadow shield is not recommended for gonad protection during fluoroscopic procedures. It has a major advantage of use in a sterile field or on incapacitated patients.

Shaped contact shields. The shaped contact shield (see Fig. 9-4) consists of a radiopaque material which is contoured to enclose the testicles. They are commonly available and can be cleaned and reused. Also available are special athletic supporters or jockey style briefs, either disposable or washable, which are used to hold the shield. The patient, within the privacy of the dressing room, can place the shaped contact shield over the penis and testicles and secure it in place by the athletic supporter or jockey style briefs. This type of shield can be effectively used during lateral and oblique projections as well as AP views. Since the shield is secured in place it can also be used during selected fluoroscopic procedures. A disadvantage of this type of shield is that problems may arise when used in sterile fields or with incapacitated patients.

Use of Gonad Shielding   Gonad shielding should be used if

   1   The gonads lie within the primary x-ray field, or within close proximity (about 5 cm) despite proper beam limitation.
   2   The clinical objectives of the examination will not be compromised.
   3   The patient has a reasonable reproductive potential.[1]

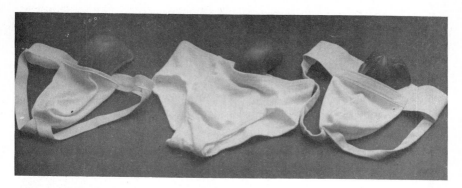

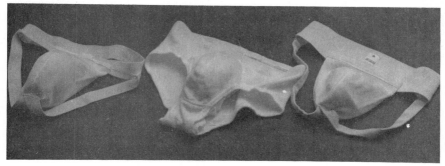

Figure 9-4 Shaped contact shields. (Bureau of Radiological Health, Food and Drug Administration, U.S. Department of Health, Education and Welfare.)

Shields should be used on patients if the gonads lie in or are in close proximity (about 5 cm) to the x-ray beam and if they *do not interfere with the objectives of the examination.*

The following are examples of where male gonad shielding may interfere with the objectives of the examination:[8]

Retrograde urethrograms
Voiding cystourethrograms
Oblique views of the hips
Visualization of the rectum
Pubic symphysis (occasionally may interfere)

The following are examples for which male gonad shielding, in the absence of extenuating circumstances, should always be used:[8]

Pelvis
Hip (except oblique views)
Upper femur

Other examinations where the testes usually are not excluded from the x-ray field by collimation alone, using conventional techniques.

Proper Filtration   Proper filtration preferentially removes lower-energy photons from the primary x-ray beam. These low-energy photons would have primarily interacted with the patient's tissues and would not have appreciably contributed to the radiographic image. Instead, they will, in the diagnostic x-ray range, increase the patient's skin dose. Therefore, filtration (usually, in the diagnostic x-ray range, aluminum) is added as required to diagnostic x-ray equipment. The amount of total filtration required depends upon the kilovolts peak of the unit and is expressed in the federal x-ray performance standard for certified equipment as a minimum half-value layer (HVL) at various kVps.

Optimum kVp Techniques   As the kVp is increased, the average energy of the x-ray photons is also increased. This means that the probability of interaction by the photoelectric effect in the patient's tissue has decreased (see Chap. 1). The decrease in tissue interactions leads to a decrease in the patient's skin dose.

Since subject contrast is decreasing with increased kVp (see Chap. 7), there is an optimum kVp for a procedure with a particular image-receptor system. Further increases in kVp can lead to poor subject contrast or too long a gray scale.

Although increased kVp does decrease the patient's skin dose, the higher-energy photons that are scattered internally (and the released electrons) can travel further prior to their complete interaction with the tissues of the body. This results in a slight, but measurable, increase in internal organ dose. The consensus is that while kVp does slightly increase internal organ dose, it is more than compensated by the marked reduction in patient skin dose.

High-Speed Image-Receptor System   The fastest possible image-receptor system *consistent with good diagnostic results* should be used. A high-speed system, even though it will reduce patient dose, cannot be used in all situations because of a loss of radiographic image quality. The selection of the proper film-screen combination to be used for a specific radiographic procedure requires a knowledge of their combined sensitivity. The radiologic technologist can ask the respective manufacturers or distributors if such information is available for their particular products.

Proper Darkroom Procedure

Darkroom Itself A radiologic technologist should ascertain if the darkroom is dark. Many darkrooms are not dark, in that there are light leaks around doors or windows. Another source of extraneous light in a darkroom is leaks from cracked or deteriorated safelight filters. In addition, the newer green-sensitive x-ray films require limits of the safelight wattage used in various filter systems.

It is suggested that the radiologic technologist test a darkroom for both external light leaks and/or safelight problems by:

1   Exposing a radiographic film such that it has a density of approximately one.
2   Keeping the undeveloped film in a lighttight envelope, in the dark darkroom pull out about one-sixth of the film for approximately 10 sec; then pull out another one-sixth of the film for approximately 10 sec.
3   Do this for a total of 6 times or approximately 60 sec such that one-sixth of the film has had about a 60-sec exposure in the darkroom, while the final one-sixth has had only about a 10-second exposure.
4   Develop the film.
5   If there are any noticeable density stripes on the film, the darkroom is not dark and steps should be taken to correct the situation.

A darkroom that is not dark can result in increased film fog and decreased radiographic detail, and could require a retake with increased patient exposure.

Manufacturer Recommendations Develop all radiographic film according to the time-temperature recommendations of the manufacturer. If it is not possible to use the film and developer (chemistry) from the same manufacturer, the radiologic technologist should ask the local chemical representative if his company has determined optimum processing conditions for the particular film that is being used. For manual processing this could take as long as 5 min at 20°C (68°F) for the maximum contrast to be developed. All darkrooms should have timers and a developer solution thermometer.

If the radiograph, developed following full manufacturer recommendations, is too dark, the film and the patient have been overexposed. If a retake is necessary, one or more of the machine settings must be changed. Do not attempt to compensate for overexposure by underdevelopment. Underdevelopment does not permit the maximum slope of the *H* and *D* curve to be formed. This results in decreased density difference (decreased contrast) and therefore a less than optimum radiograph.

In situations such as the operating room where radiographs may be needed as soon as possible, either an automatic processor should be available or the installation should utilize a commercial self-developing film process.

Automatic processors require regular maintenance. It is also specifically recommended that the rollers be kept clean. Test films of known visible light exposure should be periodically developed in order to ascertain if there have been any changes in optical densities caused by the processor. A relatively simple and inexpensive light source for exposing film has been described by E. Dale Trout.[9] Because of the problem of exact reproducibility of x-ray exposures from diagnostic units, radiographic step wedges are *not* adequate to check uniformity of processors. In order to have processor uniformity, the manufacturer's instructions as to flow rate and temperature should be followed. Since mercury contamination of the processor could occur if a glass thermometer broke, it is suggested that only metal-stemmed thermometers be used.

Since developing solutions are alkaline reducing agents, they will interact with the oxygen in air. Therefore only fresh solutions should be used. All developing solutions in storage should be kept tightly sealed.

Methods to Minimize Operator Exposure

All of the above six methods to minimize patient exposure also assist in minimizing operator exposure.

Proper collimation. As the size of the beam is decreased, the total number of photons which can undergo Compton scatter is also decreased. Therefore, proper collimation leads to minimizing the dose to the operator from scattered x-rays.

Gonad shielding. The concept of shielding can be extended to lead aprons or shielded barriers which decrease operator exposure.

Proper filtration. Filtration removes the lower-energy photons from the primary x-ray beam. These low-energy photons interact with the patient's tissues both by the photoelectric effect and by Compton scatter. The low-energy photons that would have interacted by Compton scatter could theoretically also increase operator dose. However, proper filtration removes most of these photons within the collimator so they do not have the opportunity to externally scatter.

Optimum kVp techniques. As the average energy of the photons is increased by increasing kVp, the probability of more forward scatter (rather than backscatter) is also increased (see Chap. 1). Therefore, as the kVp is increased, with a corresponding decrease in mAs, the total quantity of backscattered radiation is also decreased.

High-speed receptor system. As the speed of the receptor system is increased the "on" time of the unit is decreased. This results in fewer x-ray photons that are available for Compton scatter. If fewer photons are scattered, the operator's dose is also decreased.

Darkroom. If the darkroom is dark, and if proper development procedures are used, there will be fewer repeats and therefore less scatter exposure to the operator. If the radiograph is of optimum diagnostic quality, then it has been properly exposed, the patient has not been overexposed, and the operator has not been needlessly exposed.

In summary, the methods that the radiologic technologist uses to minimize patient dose also minimize operator dose.

In addition to the above techniques to minimize operator exposure, the following methods should also be utilized to *further* reduce operator exposure.

Shielded Booth   The operator should stand entirely within the shielded booth when using fixed radiographic equipment. Since the eyes are also a critical organ (see Chap. 5), it is important that the operator's head be behind the shielded booth. The operator should use either the lead-equivalent glass or a mirror system to view the patient.

Every time x-rays scatter, the intensity at 90° and 1 m from the scattering object is decreased by a factor of approximately 1,000. Therefore, if the exposure in the primary beam is 1,000 mR, the exposure at 90° and 1 m from the scattering object is about 1 mR. In order to minimize operator exposure, no x-rays should enter the shielded booth unless they have been scattered at least twice. This means that if the distance factor is ignored, the intensity of the x-rays in the shielded booth is only about $1/_{1,000} \times 1/_{1,000}$ or approximately $1/_{1,000,000}$ of the primary beam.

Exposure Cord Length   For fixed radiographic units, the cord should be short in order to require the operator to be behind the leaded booth during x-ray exposures.

Holding Patients   No person should be used routinely to hold a film or patients. On those occasions when it is necessary to hold a patient, the individual should be protected as far as practicable from the primary beam. This includes a leaded apron and if appropriate, leaded gloves. In addition, special instructions should be given to the holder such as to stay as far as possible out of the primary beam. To assist in minimizing exposure it is very important for the radiologic technologist to carefully collimate to the area of clinical interest.

Personnel Monitoring   Film badges, TLDs, or pocket dosimeters are recommended for use by operators of medical x-ray equipment. When a leaded apron is worn, the monitoring device shall be worn *outside* the leaded apron at the collar.[2] This procedure will approximate the dose to the eyes which as critical organs have the same maximum permissible dose equivalent as whole body or gonads (see Chap. 5).

It is also important that the operator be consistent as to where the device is worn in order that any exposure reading be properly interpreted. If more than one device is used, each dose shall be identified with the area where the device was worn on the body.

Even though monitoring-device exposures may be negative or very small, the report can act as a quality control check for the operator. If either over a period of time, the periodic reports indicate a trend of increasing exposure, or if there is a sudden marked increase, the operator and/or supervisor should attempt to ascertain the reason(s) for the increase.

Special Requirements for Mobile Equipment

a   The exposure cord for mobile equipment should be of sufficient length to permit the operator to be at least 12 ft from the tube head assembly during an exposure.[2] An exception to this is if the console itself can act as a massive barrier. In this case, the exposure switch should be extremely short or part of the console.

b   All operators of mobile equipment should wear a leaded apron along with a personnel monitoring device.

c   Since x-rays in the diagnostic x-ray range have a minimum intensity at a scatter angle of 90° (see Chap. 1), the best place for the operator to stand *if all other factors are equal* is at right angles to the scattering object. This is illustrated in Fig. 9-5.

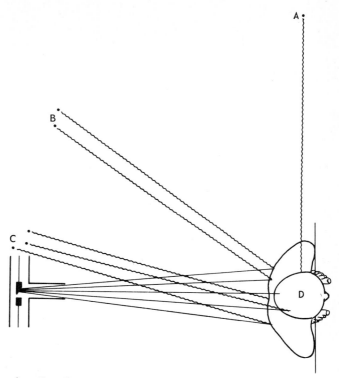

Figure 9-5   Intensity of scattered x-rays.

Assume in Fig. 9-5 that the distance $\overline{AD}$ is the same as $\overline{BD}$ or $\overline{CD}$. If all other factors are equal then the diagnostic x-ray operator will receive the minimum scatter exposure standing at position A. The maximum scatter exposure will be received at position C because of the backscatter from the patient.

The term *all other factors being equal* refers to protection factors such as distance and shielding being equal. However, if the operator can stand at a position which is further away from the scattering object than at right angles, he should consider doing so in order to utilize the protection factor of distance (inverse-square law).

The same concept is also true for shielding. If the operator does not have a protective barrier at right angles to the scattering object but does have one at a different position, he should stand behind the shield. However, if all other factors are equal the diagnostic x-ray operator will receive a minimum exposure at right angles to the scattering object.

FLUOROSCOPIC UNITS

Depending upon the state regulations or if it is certified to meet the federal x-ray performance standard, some fluoroscopic units may have an exposure rate as high as 10 R/min. If an optional high-level control is used during recording of the images, the exposure rate can be even higher. When the high-level controls are being used, a continuous signal audible to the fluoroscopist shall be activated. In addition, special means shall be utilized to avoid the accidental use of the high-level control. This can be accomplished by the requirement of additional pressure applied continuously by the operator.

All personnel not within a shielded booth shall wear a leaded apron and a personnel monitoring device. Because of the potentially high scatter exposure rate, all personnel in the room should utilize the protection devices of time, distance, or shielding. The unit shall be on for the shortest period of time consistent with the examination. Individuals not directly involved with a particular procedure should either be in a shielded control booth or as far as possible from the fluoroscopic table. This is especially important during image recording such as cine radiography or when high-level controls are being used.

The 1974 draft revision of the "Suggested State Regulations for Control of Radiation"[2] states that

> No portion of any staff or ancillary person's body, except the extremities, shall be exposed to the unattenuated scattered radiation emanating from above the tabletop unless that individual is at least 120 cm. from the center of the useful beam, or the radiation has passed through not less than 0.25 mm. lead equivalent material (e.g., drapes, Bucky-slot cover, sliding or folding panel or self supporting curtains) in addition to any lead equivalency provided by the protective apron, [(0.25 mm. minimum). Exceptions to the above suggested regulation] may be made in some special procedures where a sterile field will not permit the use of the normal protective barriers.[2]

QUESTIONS

9-1   Give three reasons why proper collimation is so important.
9-2   What should be the dimensions of a lead collimator which is inserted 3 in from the x-ray source (target) if the fixed SID is 36 in and a beam size of 8 × 10 in is required?
9-3   What type of gonad shield is best suited for use in a sterile field?
9-4   Why, in your opinion, are gonad shields not widely used?

9-5   As kVp is increased (and mAs correspondingly decreased to maintain radiographic density), what happens to
a Patient skin dose?
b Patient internal organ dose?
c Radiographic contrast?

9-6   If a child must be held during a radiographic procedure, what precautions should the holder take? Should the operator routinely hold patients?

9-7   According to your personnel monitoring records, what has been your exposure during the past six months? What do you have in your rem bank account?

9-8   In order to receive the minimum exposure, all other factors being equal, where should the operator stand during a mobile radiographic procedure on a recumbent patient?

9-9   If the tabletop exposure rate of a fluoroscope is 10 R/min, approximate the exposure rate at 90°, 1 m from a scattering object.

9-10   If upon development by an automatic processor the radiograph is too dark, what would you do?

REFERENCES

1   "Gonad Shielding in Diagnostic Radiology," U.S. Department of Health, Education and Welfare, Public Health Service, Food and Drug Administration, DHEW Publication (FDA) 75-8024, June 1975.

2   "Suggested State Regulations for Control of Radiation," Draft for Clearance through the Council of State Governments, December 30, 1974.

3   "Low Dosage Medical Roentgenography," Indiana State Board of Health, Indiana University Medical Center, Department of Radiology, 1964.

4   "We Want You to Know About Diagnostic X-Rays," U.S. Department of Health, Education, and Welfare, Public Health Service, Food and Drug Administration, DHEW Publication (FDA) 73-8048, 1974.

5   NCRP: Basic Radiation Protection Criteria, *NCRP Report* 39, NCRP Publications, 1971.

6   NCRP: Medical X-Ray and Gamma-Ray Protection for Energies up to 10 MeV, *NCRP Report* 34, NCRP Publications, 1968.

7   "Variability in the Automatic Processing of Medical X-Ray Film," U.S. DHEW, Public Health Service, Bureau of Radiological Health, BRH/DEP 70-13, 1970.

8   Proposed Rules, Specific Area Gonad Shielding, Guideline for Use on Patients During Medical Diagnostic X-Ray Procedures, Federal Register, vol. 40, no. 180, 42749, September 16, 1975.

9   Trout, E. D., et al.: A System for Periodic Testing of Film Processing, *Radiol. Technol.*, vol. 43, no. 1, July 1971.

Chapter 10

United States Governmental Radiation Control

Objectives

To provide the reader with a basic understanding of governmental regulations concerning human use x-ray equipment standards. The student should

    1 Be able to discuss the traditional state and federal roles in terms of radiation control
    2 Understand the rationale of the Council of State Governments' "Suggested State Regulations for Control of Radiation"
    3 Be aware of the current jurisdiction of state and federal activities as they pertain to ionizing radiation used in the healing arts
    4 Be able to discuss the federal x-ray standards which are relevant to radiologic technologists

STATE AND FEDERAL ACTIVITIES

State Radiation Control

While radiation safety ultimately lies with the user, some governmental control appears necessary. Under the Constitution, the ultimate responsibility in the United States for most aspects of health protection—including radiological health—is vested in the states. Traditionally the states have accepted this responsibility and are protecting the health of their citizens through their basic public health law and by specific laws concerning specialized fields, e.g., radiological health and occupational health.

By the prudent use of these laws and associated regulations, the states have for many years been engaged in effective radiological health activities such as nuclear environmental surveillance, fallout measurements, radium and x-ray control, radiation user educational programs, and radiation emergency responses. An excellent example of a state action which involved the public health is the outright banning by the individual states of shoe-fitting fluoroscopes. These fluoroscopes served no useful purpose and were a source of high radiation exposure to the unsuspecting consumer.

Having compatible regulations between states is as desirable in radiological health as it is in the field of commerce. In order to standardize as far as practicable the radiation control regulations in the states, the Councils of State Governments initially published in 1962 the first "Suggested State Regulations for Control of Radiation." The U.S. Atomic Energy Commission and the Bureau of Radiological Health (BRH), U.S. Public Health Service advised and assisted in the suggested state regulations.* The early x-ray regulations were based for the most part on recognized voluntary National Standards such as the National Bureau of Standards Handbook, Number 76. Many states substantially adapted these suggested model regulations.

In 1964, 1966, and 1970, the suggested state regulations for the control of radiation were revised and updated. Most of the 1970 revisions for radiation-producing machines were based on the guidelines of appropriate publications of the National Council on Radiation Protection and Measurements (NCRP).

The suggested regulations were again revised in 1974, in order to be consistent with the Federal Radiation Control for Health and Safety Act of 1968 (PL-90-602) and amendments to the AEC regulations (Title 10 CFR). In order to keep the suggested regulations current, task forces consisting of cooperating state and federal personnel have been established in the various components of radiation safety. These task forces will propose periodic revisions (as required) to specific sections of the model.

To facilitate mutual assistance and cooperation between the states and

* In 1971, the Bureau of Radiological Health was transferred within the Public Health Service to the Food and Drug Administration. In 1974 the regulatory functions of the U.S. Atomic Energy Commission were transferred to a new agency, the Nuclear Regulatory Commission.

the various agencies of the federal government, a National Conference of Radiation Control Program Directors was established in 1968. The purpose of the Conference is to promote radiological health in all aspects and phases; to coordinate radiological health activities of governmental agencies; to encourage the interchange of experience among radiation control program directors; and to collect and make accessible to all radiation control program directors in official administrative positions such information and data as might be of assistance to them in the proper fulfillment of their duties. One of many examples of the state-federal partnership which is a direct result of this conference is the ongoing "Nationwide Evaluation of X-Ray Trends" (NEXT) program. The primary objective of NEXT is the production of meaningful, timely information for planning and evaluating x-ray control programs at the state, regional, and national levels. In this program, state x-ray inspectors, using special test methods developed by a task force of the conference and the Bureau of Radiological Health, Food and Drug Administration, are able to measure important factors which influence patient dose such as collimation, exposure, half-value layer, and time. A computer calculates the exposure as well as other important parameters and returns the information to the respective state, which can use the data to set work priorities to further minimize unnecessary radiation exposure.

Working cooperatively with the various professional societies, many states are also involved with educational programs on radiation protection. These include but are not limited to such activities as special seminars, pamphlets, books, and lectures in schools of radiologic technology.

Source by-product materials (radioisotopes obtained by the fission of uranium, thorium, or plutonium) are, unless delegated to a state through an agreement with the federal government, under the control (in terms of licensing and inspection of the facility) of the federal Nuclear Regulatory Commission. However, naturally occurring isotopes such as radium or machine-produced (accelerator) isotopes are under the direct control of the state itself.

Several states also have minimum standards for the training and education of radiologic technologists.

The reader should contact his State Radiological Health Program for any questions concerning state laws or regulations. For convenience, a list of the State Radiological Health Programs can be found in the Appendix.

Federal Activities

The U.S. Atomic Energy Commission (now the Nuclear Regulatory Commission) has since 1948 controlled source by-product materials for medical or industrial use. Many states have signed an agreement with the Nuclear Regulatory Commission by which the jurisdiction for licensing and inspection of the facilities which use by-product materials has been transferred from federal to state jurisdiction.

Federal responsibility for nonnuclear radiation control in the healing arts and consumer areas rests with the Department of Health, Education and Welfare. Traditionally, HEW's role in radiation control had been that of assistance to states, research, and public information.

With the passage of the Radiation Control for Health and Safety Act of 1968, PL-90-602, on October 8, 1968, the federal role was greatly expanded. It now includes not only the previous activities, but also the authority to set equipment performance standards of electronic products that emit electronic product radiation *if* the Secretary of the U.S. Department of Health, Education, and Welfare determines that there could be a potential health hazard to the American public. The day-to-day operations pertaining to PL-90-602 have been delegated to the Director, Bureau of Radiological Health, Food and Drug Administration, Rockville, Maryland 20852.

It is important to note that currently (1976) the Radiation Control for Health and Safety Act of 1968 only permits the federal government jurisdiction concerning the manufacture of electronic products (performance standards) and is silent as to the actual use of the product by an individual. The use of these products remains under the jurisdiction of the states.

HUMAN USE X-RAY EQUIPMENT STANDARDS

Radiation Control for Health and Safety Act of 1968 (PL-90-602)

Under PL-90-602, performance standards for human use x-ray equipment were promulgated as of August 1, 1974 by the Food and Drug Administration. This means that as of that date, it is illegal to manufacture for use in the United States any x-ray equipment for which there is a standard unless the equipment manufacturer certifies that it meets the applicable performance standard. The equipment manufacturer also attaches a permanent easily identified label to the various certifiable components of the x-ray equipment stating that it is in compliance with the standard.

In general, human use x-ray equipment manufactured prior to August 1, 1974 is under the jurisdiction of the states and as such is subject to the individual requirements of each state's regulations. However, for certified x-ray equipment, that is, human use x-ray equipment manufactured after August 1, 1974, as stated in Section 360F of the Radiation Control for Health and Safety, Act of 1968 (PL-90-602), "No state or political subdivision in a state shall have any authority either to establish or to continue in effect any standard which is applicable to the same aspect of performance of an electronic product for which there is a Federal Standard unless the State regulation is identical to the Federal Standard."

In effect this means that for the near future two sets of standards exist which may be applied to x-ray equipment depending on its date of manufacture, state and/or federal. Although many aspects of the two standards are similar, the reader should contact his state radiological health program for the specific requirements in his locality. In general, they are based on recent revisions of the Council of State Governments, "Suggested Stated Regulations for Control of Radiation."

As mentioned earlier, PL-90-602 allows federal jurisdiction concerning the certification by manufacturers on human use x-ray equipment. Since PL-90-602 defines an assembler as a manufacturer, he must also certify to the Food and Drug Administration that the unit has been assembled according to the instructions of the component manufacturer, that certified components of the type called for in the standard were used, and that other requirements have been completed. If he is engaged in the business of assembling, replacing, or installing one or more components into an x-ray system or subsystem, a radiologic technologist is considered an assembler. As such, he has the same legal obligations of an assembler.

If, following inspection by a state and/or federal inspector, a certified x-ray machine is found to be in noncompliance with the performance standard, a further investigation is initiated to find out if the reason for the noncompliance is due to either:

1   Improper equipment manufacture
2   Improper assembly
3   Improper maintenance or abuse by the user

If the reason for the noncompliance is due to either improper equipment manufacture or assembly, the responsible company must according to PL-90-602, following concurrence of the Bureau of Radiological Health, FDA:

1   Repair the unit at no charge to the owner
2   Replace the unit with one that is in compliance
3   Refund to the owner the cost of the item

If the noncompliance is due to user abuser or to not following the maintenance schedule which the manufacturer is required to provide the owner, then the federal government has no authority to require correction. However, the state radiological health programs under their laws and regulations can require the owner to make the necessary corrections to bring the unit into compliance.

Major Provisions of the Federal Human Use X-Ray Performance Standards

There are currently over 60 individual requirements of the federal x-ray performance standard. The ones that the radiologic technologist should have knowledge of in their day-to-day operations can be classified into three general areas: (1) x-ray controls, (2) fluoroscopic imaging assemblies, and (3) beam-limiting devices.

1. X-Ray Controls

   a   The technique factors used during an exposure shall be indicated before the exposure begins, except when using automatic exposure controls. This indication shall be visible from the operator's position, except for spot films.
   b   The control panel will conspicuously have the label "WARNING: This x-ray unit may be dangerous to patient and operator unless safe exposure factors and operating instructions are observed."
   c   When using automatic exposure control, if an exposure has been terminated by the backup timer, an indication shall be made on the control panel. Manual resetting is required before making further automatically timed exposures, so that the operator will know something is wrong.
   d   The x-ray control shall provide visual indication whenever x-rays are produced. An audible signal shall indicate the termination of exposure.
   e   For multiple tubes controlled by one exposure switch, the tube or tubes selected shall be clearly indicated, both at the control panel and or near the tube selected.
   f   Except during serial radiography, it shall be possible to end the exposure at any time during an exposure greater than ½ second. In serial radiography the user can complete any single exposure of a series. End of exposure shall cause automatic resetting of timer to zero or its initial setting. You cannot make an exposure when the timer is set to zero or "off".
   g   The radiation output must be linear between adjacent mA settings, i.e., output increases in proportion to the increase in mA as well as being reproducible.

2. Fluoroscopic Imaging Assemblies

   a   X-rays shall not be produced unless a primary barrier intercepts the entire useful beam. If it does not, then production of x-rays is prevented by an interlock.

b   X-ray production must be controlled by a continuous pressure device.
c   When the unit is in its high output mode, a continuous audible signal must be heard.
d   X-ray tube potential (kVp) and current (mA) shall be continuously indicated.
e   The following minimum x-ray tube to target distance shall exist:

Stationary units. . . . . .38 cm
Mobile units . . . . .30 cm
Special units . . . . .20 cm

f   The maximum cumulative time for tube exposure shall not exceed five minutes without resetting. A signal must indicate the completion of the time and it will remain on until time is reset.
g   Mobile units require intensified imaging.

3. Beam-Limiting Devices

a   In general, there must be some means of restricting the dimensions of the x-ray field. Other provisions are:

visually defining the perimeter of the field
indication when the axis of the beam is perpendicular to the plane of the image receptor
general purpose systems shall be capable of operation such that the field size at the image receptor can be smaller than the image receptor
beam limiting device shall numerically indicate the field size to which it is adjusted in inches or centimeters.

b   Means shall be provided for positive beam limitation (PBL) on stationary general purpose units which will either cause automatic adjustment of the field to the image receptor size within a certain time period or prevent production of x-rays until adjustment is completed.
c   PBL may be by-passed under certain conditions; however, when these conditions cease, return to PBL shall be automatic.
d   It is possible to override PBL by means of a key; however, it shall be impossible to remove key in override.
e   There are beam limiting requirements for spot film equipment which allows for a smaller adjustment of the field size in plane of film than the size of the film which has been selected on the spot film selector. Also, the size of the x-ray beam must be automatically limited to the size of the portion of the spot film selected *before* the beam enters the patient.*

For further information concerning the federal x-ray standard and specific legal requirements, the reader should contact the office of the appropriate Regional Radiological Health Representative, U.S. Food and Drug Ad-

---

* "What the x-ray technologist should know about the x-ray performance standard," handout literature, Bureau of Radiological Health, Food and Drug Administration, 1974.

ministration. A list of these offices and the states in their regions is provided for your convenience in the Appendix.

QUESTIONS

10-1 List several traditional roles of both state and federal government radiation control agencies.

10-2 What is one of the main purposes of the Council of State Governments "Suggested State Regulations for Control of Radiation"?

10-3 What federal agency has jurisdiction concerning performance standards for certified human use x-ray equipment?

10-4 If a certified component of an x-ray machine is found to be in noncompliance, explain the options available to the manufacturer under PL-90-602.

10-5 What agency has jurisdiction concerning the use of certified x-ray equipment?

10-6 What actions can be contemplated by the federal government if the reason for noncompliance is found to be the improper following of the maintenance schedule by the owner?

10-7 Under the federal x-ray performance standard, what is required at the x-ray control to verify that x-rays are being produced? What shall indicate the termination of exposure?

10-8 What is the maximum cumulative time for tube exposure on a fluoroscope? What happens at the end of this time?

10-9 Is a positive beam-limiting device (PBL) required on certified portable x-ray equipment? Explain your answer.

10-10 What are your state requirements concerning beam size for uncertified x-ray equipment (manufactured prior to August 1, 1974)?

REFERENCES

1 "Radiation Control for Health and Safety Act of 1968," PL-90-602 (42 U.S.C. 263n).*

2 "Regulations for the Administration and Enforcement of the Radiation Control for Health and Safety Act of 1968," U.S. Department of Health, Education, and Welfare, Public Health Service, Food and Drug Administration, DHEW Publication No. (FDA) 75-8003, 1974.*

3 "A Practitioner's Guide to the Diagnostic X-Ray Equipment Standard," U.S. Department of Health, Education, and Welfare, Public Health Service, Food and Drug Administration, DHEW Publication No. (FDA) 75-8005, 1974.*

4 Council of State Governments: "Suggested State Regulations for Control of Radiation," 1974.

   * Available through the office of the appropriate Regional Radiological Health Representative, FDA. (See Appendix for locations.)

Appendix

State, Regional, and International Radiation Control Program Directors[1]

UNITED STATES

States

Alabama

Director
Division of Radiological Health
State Department of Public Health
State Office Building
Montgomery, Alabama 36104

Alaska

Assistant Chief
Environmental Health Section
Department of Environmental Health
Pouch H-06F
Juneau, Alaska 99811

Arizona

Executive Director
Arizona Atomic Energy Commission
1601 West Jefferson Street
Phoenix, Arizona 85007

Arkansas
                Director
                Bureau of Environmental Health Services
                Department of Health
                4815 West Markham Street
                Little Rock, Arkansas 72201

California
                Chief
                Radiologic Health Section
                Health Protection Systems
                Department of Health
                Building #8
                714 P Street
                Sacramento, California 95814

                Director
                Bureau of Occupational & Radiation Management
                County of Los Angeles Department of Health Services
                Community Health Services
                Radiological Health Division
                313 North Figueroa Street
                Los Angeles, California 90012

Colorado
                Director
                Division of Occupational & Radiological Health
                Department of Health
                4210 East 11th Avenue
                Denver, Colorado 80220

Connecticut
                Assistant Director of Compliance
                Department of Environmental Protection
                State Office Building
                Hartford, Connecticut 06115

Delaware
                Program Director
                Office of Radiation Safety
                Division of Public Health
                Department of Health & Social Services
                Jesse S. Cooper Memorial Building
                Capitol Square
                Dover, Delaware 19901

District of Columbia
                Chief
                Bureau of Institutional Hygiene and Radiological Health, EHA
                Department of Environmental Services
                801 N. Capitol Street, N.W.
                Washington, D.C. 20003

Florida

Administrator
Radiological & Occupational Health Section
Division of Health
Department of Health & Rehabilitative Services
P.O. Box 210
Jacksonville, Florida 32201

Georgia

Director
Radiological Health Unit
Department of Human Resources
State Office Building
47 Trinity Avenue
Atlanta, Georgia 30334

Hawaii

Chief
Noise and Radiation Branch
Department of Health
P.O. Box 3378
Honolulu, Hawaii 96801

Idaho

Chief
Radiation Control Section
Idaho Department of Health and Welfare
Statehouse
Boise, Idaho 83720

Illinois

Chief
Division of Radiological Health
Department of Public Health
535 West Jefferson Street
Springfield, Illinois 62761

Indiana

Director
Division of Radiological Health
Indiana State Board of Health
1330 West Michigan Street
Indianapolis, Indiana 46206

Iowa

Radiation Activities
Department of Environmental Quality
3920 Delaware Street
P.O. Box 3326
Des Moines, Iowa 50316

Kansas

Director
Bureau of Radiation Control
Department of Health and Environment
Topeka, Kansas 66620

Kentucky

Manager
Radiation and Control Branch
Department for Human Resources
Capitol Annex
Frankfort, Kentucky 40601

Louisiana

Administrator
Division of Radiation Control
Natural Resources and Energy
Department of Conservation
P.O. Box 44033
Capitol Station
Baton Rouge, Louisiana 70804

Maine

Radiological Health Program Director
Department of Health and Welfare
State House
Augusta, Maine 04330

Maryland

Chief
Division of Radiation Control
Department of Health and Mental Hygiene
O'Conor Office Building
201 West Preston Street
Baltimore, Maryland 21201

Massachusetts

Assistant to the Commissioner (Radiological Health)
Massachusetts Department of Public Health
80 Boylston Street, Room 835
Boston, Massachusetts 02116

Michigan

Chief
Radiation Division
Department of Public Health
3500 North Logan Street
Lansing, Michigan 48914

Minnesota

Chief
Section of Radiation Control
Department of Health
717 Delaware Street, S.E.
Minneapolis, Minnesota 55440

Mississippi

Director
Division of Radiological Health
State Board of Health
Felix J. Underwood State Board of Health Building
P.O. Box 1700
Jackson, Mississippi 39205

Missouri

Director
Bureau of Radiological Health
Department of Social Services
2511 Industrial Drive
Jefferson City, Missouri 65101

Montana

Chief
Radiological and Occupational Health Program
Department of Health & Environmental Sciences
Cogswell Building
Helena, Montana 59601

Nebraska

Director
Division of Radiological Health
Department of Health
1003 "O" Street
Lincoln Building
Lincoln, Nebraska 68508

Nevada

Supervisor
Radiological Health
State Department of Health and Welfare
201 South Fall Street
Carson City, Nevada 89701

New Hampshire

Director
State Radiation Control Agency
State Laboratory Building
Hazen Drive
Concord, New Hampshire 03301

New Jersey

Chief
Bureau of Radiation Protection
Division of Environmental Quality
Department of Environmental Protection
380 Scotch Road
Ewing Township
Trenton, New Jersey 08628

New Mexico

Director
Environmental Improvement Agency
State of New Mexico
P.O. Box 2348
Santa Fe, New Mexico 87501

New York   Director
                                        Bureau of Radiological Health
                                        Community Health Services
                                        Empire State Plaza
                                        Tower Building
                                        Albany, New York 12237

                                        Director
                                        Bureau of Radiologic Technology*
                                        Health Manpower Group
                                        Empire State Plaza
                                        Tower Building
                                        Albany, New York 12237

                                        Director
                                        Office of Radiation Control
                                        New York City Department of Health
                                        325 Broadway
                                        New York, New York 10007

North Carolina   Head
                                        Radiation Protection Branch
                                        Division of Facility Services
                                        Department of Human Resources
                                        P.O. Box 12200
                                        Raleigh, North Carolina 27605

North Dakota   Director
                                        Division of Environmental Engineering
                                        North Dakota State Department of Health
                                        Capitol Building
                                        Bismarck, North Dakota 58501

Ohio   Engineer-in-Charge
                                        Radiological Health Unit
                                        Department of Health
                                        P.O. Box 118
                                        Columbus, Ohio 43216

Oklahoma   Chief
                                        Occupational & Radiological Health Service
                                        State Department of Health
                                        N.E. 10th and Stonewall Streets
                                        P.O. Box 53551
                                        Oklahoma City, Oklahoma 73105

* User certification only.

Oregon

Director
Radiation Control Service
State Health Division
P.O. Box 231
Portland, Oregon 97207

Pennsylvania

Director
Pennsylvania Bureau of Radiological Health
Department of Environmental Resources
P.O. Box 2063
Harrisburg, Pennsylvania 17120

Chief
Occupational & Radiological Health Section
Environmental Health Services
Philadelphia Department of Public Health
500 South Broad Street
Philadelphia, Pennsylvania 19146

Puerto Rico

Director
Radiological Health Program
Department of Health
1306 Ponce de Leon Avenue
Stop 16
Santurce, Puerto Rico 00908

Rhode Island

Division of Occupational Health
Department of Health
Health Department Building
Davis Street
Providence, Rhode Island 02908

South Carolina

Director
Division of Radiological Health
S.C. Dept. of Health & Environmental Control
137 J. Marion Sims Building
Columbia, South Carolina 29201

South Dakota

Sanitation and Safety Program
State Department of Health
State Capitol
Pierre, South Dakota 57501

Tennessee

Director
Division of Occupational & Radiological Health
Department of Public Health
727 Cordell Hull Building
Sixth Avenue, North
Nashville, Tennessee 27219

Texas   Director
                             Division of Occupational Health & Radiation Control
                             Texas Department of Health Resources
                             1100 West 49th Street
                             Austin, Texas 78756

Utah   Chief
                             Radiation & Occupational Health Section
                             State Division of Health
                             44 Medical Drive
                             Salt Lake City, Utah 84113

Vermont   Director
                             Division of Occupational Health
                             Radiological Health Program
                             Department of Health
                             P.O. Box 607
                             Barre, Vermont 05641

Virginia   Director
                             Bureau of Industrial Hygiene and Radiological Health
                                 Supervisor
                             Department of Health
                             109 Governor Street
                             Richmond, Virginia 23219

Virgin Islands   Director
                             Natural Resources Management
                             Division of Natural Resources
                             Department of Conservation and Cultural Affairs
                             P.O. Box 578
                             Department of Health
                             Charlotte Amalie
                             St. Thomas, Virgin Islands 00801

Washington   Supervisor
                             Radiation Control Unit
                             Department of Social and Health Services
                             P.O. Box 1788, MS 17-1
                             Olympia, Washington 98504

West Virginia   Director
                             Bureau of Industrial Hygiene
                             Radiological Health Program
                             State Department of Health
                             1800 East Washington Street
                             Charleston, West Virginia 25305

Wisconsin   Chief
                         Radiation Protection Section
                         Department of Health & Social Services
                         P.O. Box 309
                         Madison, Wisconsin 53701

Wyoming   Chief
                         Radiological Health Services
                         Department of Health & Social Services
                         Division of Health & Medical Services
                         New State Office Building
                         Cheyenne, Wyoming 82001

Federal

US Department of Health, Education and Welfare
Public Health Service
Food and Drug Administration
Bureau of Radiological Health
5600 Fishers Lane
Rockville, Maryland 20852

US Department of Health, Education and Welfare
Public Health Service
Food and Drug Administration
Office of the Executive Director of Regional Operations
Director, Radiation Operations Staff
5600 Fishers Lane
Rockville, Maryland 20852

REGIONAL RADIOLOGICAL HEALTH REPRESENTATIVES, FDA

Region I (Conn., Maine, Mass., N.H., R.I., Vt.)

Regional Radiological Health Representative
DHEW, PHS, FDA
585 Commercial Street
Boston, Massachusetts 02109

Region II (N.J., N.Y., P.R., V.I.)

Regional Radiological Health Representative
DHEW, PHS, FDA
850 Third Avenue
Brooklyn, New York 11232

Region III (Del., D.C., Md., Pa., Va., W.Va.)

Regional Radiological Health Representative
DHEW, PHS, FDA
900 U.S. Customhouse
Second and Chestnut Streets
Philadelphia, Pennsylvania 19106

Region IV (Ala., Fla., Ga., Ky., Miss., N.C., S.C., Tenn.)

Regional Radiological Health Representative
DHEW, PHS, FDA
880 West Peachtree Street, N.W.
Atlanta, Georgia 30309

Region V (Ill., Ind., Mich., Minn., Ohio, Wis.)

Regional Radiological Health Representative
DHEW, PHS, FDA
Room A 1945
175 West Jackson Boulevard
Chicago, Illinois 60604

Region VI (Ark., La., N. Mex., Okla., Tex.)

Regional Radiological Health Representative
DHEW, PHS, FDA
Room 470B
500 South Ervay Street
Dallas, Texas 75201

Region VII (Iowa, Kans., Mo., Nebr.)

Regional Radiological Health Representative
DHEW, PHS, FDA
1009 Cherry Street
Kansas City, Missouri 64106

Region VIII (Colo., Mont., N. Dak., S. Dak., Utah, Wyo.)

Regional Radiological Health Representative
DHEW, PHS, FDA
Room 500
U.S. Customhouse
Denver, Colorado 80202

Region IX (Ariz., Calif., Hawaii, Nev., Guam, American Samoa)

Regional Radiological Health Representative
DHEW, PHS, FDA
Federal Office Building
50 Fulton Street
San Francisco, California 94102

Region X (Alaska, Idaho, Oreg., Wash.)

Regional Radiological Health Representative
DHEW, PHS, FDA
Room 5003, Federal Office Building
909 First Avenue
Seattle, Washington 98104

GREAT BRITAIN

National Radiological Protection Board,
Headquarters and Southern Centre,
Harwell,
Didcot,
Berks.

National Radiological Protection Board,
Northern Centre,
29 Clarendon Road,
Leeds. LS2 9PD

National Radiological Protection Board,
Scottish Centre,
11 West Graham Street,
Glasgow. GL4 9LF

AUSTRALIA

New South Wales
The Chairman,
Health Commission of New South Wales,
9–13 Young Street, Sydney, N.S.W. 2000

Victoria
The Secretary,
Commission of Public Health,
295 Queen Street, Melbourne, Vic. 3000

Queensland
The Director-General of Health and Medical Services,
Department of Health,
Administration Building,
63–79 George Street, Brisbane, Qld 4000

South Australia
The Director-General of Public Health,
158 Rundle Street, Adelaide, S.A. 5000

Western Australia
The Commissioner of Public Health,
Department of Public Health,
57 Murray Street, Perth, W.A. 6000

Tasmania
The Director of Public Health,
Department of Health Services,
Public Buildings, Hobart, Tas. 7000

Australian Capital Territory
The Director-General of Health,
Department of Health,
Box 100, Woden, A.C.T. 2606

Northern Territory
Director of Health,
Department of Health,
P.O. Box 147, Darwin, N.T. 5794

CANADA

Nuclear Radiation

Atomic Energy Control Board
P.O. Box 1046
Ottawa, Ont. KIP 5A9

X-Ray Radiation

Radiation Protection Service
Department of Health
Confederation Bldg.
St. John's, Newfoundland

Radiation Protection Service,
Department of Health,
P.O. Box 3000
Charlottetown, P.E.I.

Radiation Protection Service
Department of Health
Centennial Bldg.
Fredericton, N.B.

Radiation Protection Service
Department of Health
Hollis St.
Halifax, N.S.

Protection Centre Les Rayons X
Ministere des Affaires Sociales
1075 Chemin Ste Foy
Quebec, Que.

X-Ray Inspection Service
Ontario Ministry of Health
Queens Park
Toronto, Ont.

Radiation Protection Service
Department of Health & Social Development
700 Bannatyne Ave.
Winnipeg, Man.

Radiations Protection Service
Department of Public Health
Provincial Health Bldg.
Regina, Sask.

Radiation Protection Service
Department of Health & Social Development
Administration Bldg.
Edmonton, Alta.

Radiation Protection Service
Department of Health
Parliament Bldg.
Victoria, B.C.

REFERENCE

1 "Directory of Personnel Responsible for Radiological Health Programs," U.S. Department of Health, Education, and Welfare, DHEW Publication (FDA) 76-8006, July 1975.

Answers to Questions

Some of the questions in the text have more than *one* possible correct answer; that is, they are discussion questions. Therefore the response listed below for this type of question is preceded by the term *Discussion Question.*

Chapter 1

1-1   Photoelectric effect; increase.

1-2   1,020 keV (1.02 MeV); no.

1-3   No; A roentgen is defined in *air* only for x- or gamma radiation.

1-4   Barium has an atomic number or Z number of 56; The purpose of barium is to act as a radiopaque media to diagnostic x-rays. It effectively does this because its high Z number causes a high probability of the photoelectric effect; No, sodium (Z number of 11) has too low an atomic number to be radiopaque in the diagnostic x-ray range.

1-5   The probability of Compton scatter increases as the photon energy increases. In water it reaches its peak around 500 keV and then decreases.

1-6   50 rems.

1-7   5 rems.

1-8 Backscatter; If all other factors are equal, the minimum scatter angle from the scattering object will be 90°.

1-9 rad; roentgen; curie; rem.

1-10 In the diagnostic x-ray range, the predominant type of interaction is the photoelectric effect. A major factor in determining the probability of occurrence of the photoelectric effect is the atomic number or Z number. Since the Z number of lead is 82, while aluminum's is 13, lead is a more efficient shield for diagnostic x-rays.

Chapter 2

2-1 Ionizing radiation interacts with water to form free radicals which can oxidize DNA. Since aqueous free radicals are mobile, the ionizing event does not have to be directly on the DNA molecule itself.

2-2 No; Exposure to ionizing radiation can result in an irreparable component of injury. Additional exposure could lead to further irreparable injury. Therefore, contrary to the typical antigen-antibody reaction, no immunity is acquired; instead with continued exposure just the opposite, a gradual buildup of irreparable injury occurs.

2-3 Approximately 270 rads.

2-4 Blood precursor cells are (1) "simple" and (2) rapidly dividing. The theory of Bergonié and Tribondeau states that simple and rapidly dividing cells are very sensitive to ionizing radiation.

2-5 To increase the probability of formation of the free radical HO_2.

2-6 Linear (straight line); There is no threshold for genetic response.

2-7 Discussion question
a   Medical evaluation.
b   Where was the dosimeter worn, i.e., on the outside or inside of the leaded apron; at the waist or at the collar?
c   Was it partial or whole-body exposure?
d   Over what period of time was the exposure received?
e   Ascertain the cause of the exposure.

2-8 Initial, latent, manifest illness, recovery or death; No.

2-9 Hematopoietic, gastrointestinal, and central nervous system deaths.

2-10 The inhibition of production of megakaryocytes (which fragment into blood platelets when mature) prevents the proper clotting of blood.

Chapter 3

3-1 Discussion question. The probability of life-span shortening as a function of radiation exposure is statistical in nature. Therefore, if a large number of individuals were to receive a low or intermediate dose of radiation, statistically, the life span of the large group *as a whole* could be shortened. However, the probability of any one individual's life span being shortened as a result of this exposure is small.

3-2 Carcinogenesis, embryological, cataractogenesis, life-span shortening.

3-3 Not necessarily; if you are on the straight-line part of the curve, then a doubling dose could also result in a doubling of the effect.

3-4 Yes.

3-5   Since by the period of the fetus, the organs have been formed, the cells are more specialized and also not multiplying as rapidly, as during the period of major organogenesis.

3-6   Discussion question.
1   Inform supervisor and/or the radiologist prior to any retake.
2   Ascertain how, in the future, this type of situation could be avoided.

3-7   Extremely sensitive during early morphogenesis; relatively insensitive.

3-8   Malignancies of the bone. Radium which is chemically similar to calcium is concentrated in the bone.

3-9   Discussion question. If the radiation dose to x-ray operators in the United States is low, the expected numbers of their cancer mortality rate should be essentially the same as those of the public cancer mortality rate. Most diagnostic radiographic operator exposures are quite low. However, this may not necessarily be the case of improperly protected fluoroscopic operators.

3-10 Since radium is chemically similar to calcium, it is concentrated in the bone.

Chapter 4

4-1 $T, C, G, A; T\text{-}A, G\text{-}C$.

4-2   The basic meanings in the DNA code translate into the 20 basic amino acids.

4-3   Messenger RNA (mRNA).

4-4   The major function of the ribosomes is to synthesize proteins from the 20 basic amino acids.

4-5   If a gene leads to an enzyme that causes a specific effect to occur, it is dominant; otherwise, it is recessive.

4-6   Discussion question. We are very concerned about the possible long-term genetic effects since they may not become fully apparent until an individual is conceived who carries both recessive genes of the same trait. This may not occur until generations after the initial exposure.

4-7   A point mutation can occur resulting in the displacement of a base letter. This can lead to a word change resulting in a modified enzyme.

4-8   Discussion question. If there is no threshold, then in theory one photon could cause a mutation. In practice this would be very remote. However, as the number of photons increase, the probability of an effect also increases. Therefore, in terms of good public health practice, the exposure to all concerned should be minimized consistent with the maximum benefits derived from the radiation.

4-9   The primary function of tRNA is to serve as a carrier for the appropriate amino acid to the correct location on the mRNA.

4-10 Nucleotides are the organic base letters ($A, T, G,$ and C) attached to a sugar-phosphate base. Their function is to combine with a complementary letter on the single strand of DNA.

Chapter 5

5-1   5.0 rems.

5-2   0.1 rem.

5-3   Discussion question. The cause of the exposure should be determined and corrected, and the individual student should be carefully monitored. If the dose equivalent actually reaches 0.1 rem, the student should be removed from the educational radiation environment. Students under 18 should not be occupationally exposed to ionizing radiation. The 0.1 R per year represents radiation received during educational activities.

5-4   Discussion question. Radiation workers represent only a very small fraction of the world's population. Any deleterious somatic effects would, as a function of time, be diluted with the rest of the population.

5-5   15 rems.

5-6   Yes; No. The worker at age 21 has 15 rems less 7 rems, or 8 rems, in the bank account. During the next year, he accumulates 5 additional rems, so that at the end of the year he has $8 + 5 = 13$ rems. Therefore, he has sufficient rems in the bank account to receive 12 rems during the year. Since 12 rems were received, at the end of the year he has only $13 - 12 = 1$ rem remaining in the bank account.

During the second year, he accumulates an additional 5 rems in his bank account. This means that at the end of the second year he has $1 + 5 = 6$ rems in the bank account. Therefore, he cannot receive 12 rems during the second year, since at the end of that year only 6 rems are in his bank account.

5-7   Discussion question

1   Determine why the readings were higher than the average.

2   Based on the answer above, instruct the operator on radiation safety procedures.

The reading of 85 mR per month is not considered dangerous for an individual.

5-8   0.5 rem.

5-9   No.

5-10   Discussion question. 0.5 rem during the gestation period; If an operator says she is four months pregnant:

1   Estimate her abdominal exposure during the 4-month period.

2   Ask a health physicist or radiation physicist to estimate fetal dose.

3   Carefully monitor future exposures during her pregnancy.

4   If necessary, based on the radiation doses involved, remove her from the radiation environment.

Chapter 6

6-1   3 mR; The lower reading should be recorded since the higher reading could have been caused by accidental shock-type discharge or a short circuit due to dust or excessive moisture.

6-2   No.

6-3   *Advantages*
Fast reading
Inexpensive
Lightweight

Disadvantages
Limited range
Energy dependent
Physical shock can discharge the unit
Not a permanent record

6-4 To estimate effective energy of the beam. It is important because the density of the film is related to the energy of the beam as well as the actual exposure.

6-5 *Advantages*
Permanent record
Inexpensive
Relatively accurate if interpreted correctly
Lightweight
Disadvantages
Energy dependent
Must wait for development
Subject to environmental factors such as heat or moisture

6-6 In a TLD, an electron after receiving energy from an ionizing event is trapped in the forbidden zone. Heat raises it to a level where it can return to its normal state with the emission of a light photon. The intensity of light emitted can be correlated with initial radiation exposure.

6-7 *Advantages*
Relatively energy independent
Inexpensive
Small
Accurate
Disadvantages
Not in itself a permanent record
Fading
Must wait for results

6-8 The rate meter measures exposure (or dose or counts) per unit of time, an example would be mR/h. An integrating device determines the total exposure (or dose or counts) received.

6-9 A Geiger counter should not be used for diagnostic x-ray surveys unless it has a special probe sensitive to and calibrated in the diagnostic x-ray range.

6-10 No. The reason is that the normal "on" time of a diagnostic radiographic examination is too short for proper instrument response.

Chapter 7

7-1 3.

7-2 0.4 to more than 3.

7-3 No; A properly developed radiograph that is too dark indicates overexposure. It should be retaken using modified technique factors. Shortened development time leads to decreased contrast.

7-4 As kVp increases, the gray scale becomes longer. This is because as kVp increases, subject contrast decreases, because of a decreased ratio of exposures of adjacent tissues to the film.

7-5 Although uniform scatter may be added to a film, the amount of darkening (density) depends on the total exposure received by the film. This can be ascertained by looking at the exposure axis (x axis) of a characteristic curve and noting the large change in density per added scatter exposure at the lower part of each log cycle as compared to the same added scatter exposure at the upper part of the same cycle.

7-6 Increase; A grid removes much of the scattered radiation.

7-7 High-speed screen–film combination.

7-8 Discussion question. Slower-speed image-receptor systems generally provide greater detail visibility, but at the price of increased radiation exposure. If this quality of detail visibility is not needed for a particular examination, a higher-speed system should be used in order to reduce radiation exposure.

7-9 Graininess is the chance accumulation of developed grains. It is increased as kVp is increased because of increased photoelectron or Compton electron interactions with nearby silver halide crystals.

7-10 Discussion question. kVp, grids, collimation, film, screen, processing, mAs, SID, and motion.

Chapter 8

8-1 Discussion question. There is no one best answer. It could be time, distance, or shielding. The optimum protection factor or factors depend upon the specific situation.

8-2 6.66 h.

8-3 As filtration (or shielding) increases, the lower-energy photons of an x-ray spectrum are preferentially removed by the photoelectric effect. Therefore, the average energy of the beam increases. This means that the beam "acts" as if it were of a greater monoenergetic energy. The greater the photon energy, the greater the half-value layer.

8-4 Not necessarily; It depends on the HVL of the wood. If it were one cm; i.e., if the HVL of wood is 1 cm for the diagnostic x-rays used, then the addition of one HVL (1 cm) would decrease the exposure by 50 percent. The actual HVL of the wood depends not only on the type and density of wood but also on the energy of the beam.

8-5 1,210 mR.

8-6

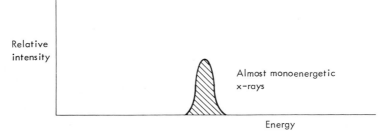

The beam is almost monoenergetic since the lower-energy photons have been removed by the photoelectric effect while passing through the lead tube housing.

8-7   Call for assistance. Know who to immediately contact in case of an emergency.

8-8   4.98 cm.

8-9   Discussion question. Ingestion, inhalation, and absorption

Ingestion: Avoid eating or smoking in areas where unsealed sources are used or stored. Monitor and wash hands prior to eating or smoking. Monitor the work area; wear appropriate gloves and protective clothing.

Inhalation: Use as required a radiation hood or glove box. If necessary, a mask or self-contained breathing apparatus can be used. Have proper air monitors. Also monitor (wipe tests) the work area.

Absorption: Avoid contamination on the skin by using appropriate gloves and protective clothing. Monitor the work area.

8-10 No; Since leaded aprons contain about 0.5 mm of lead equivalent, or much less than 1 HVL (1.66 cm), they do not safely attenuate the gamma-ray beam. However, the apron may actually increase the operator's dose by:
1   A false sense of security
2   Slows the operator's work

Chapter 9

9-1   Minimize patient exposure, decrease scattered x-rays on the film, decrease scatter exposure to the operator.

9-2   0.67 × 0.83 in.

9-3   Shadow shield.

9-4   Discussion question. Not motivated, too embarrassing, too much trouble, interferes with the examination.

9-5   a   Decreases
         b   Slightly increases
         c   Decreases

9-6   The holder should be instructed as to what to do during the procedure. He shall also wear a leaded apron and if possible leaded gloves. The individual shall also be specifically instructed to stay as far from the useful beam as possible. The radiologic technologist must collimate to the specific area of clinical interest; No.

9-7   Individual project question.

9-8   At right angles or 90° to the scattering object.

9-9   Approximately 10 mR/min or 600 mR/h.

9-10 Modify the radiographic techniques to reduce the exposure. The processor should also routinely be checked for proper functioning.

Chapter 10

10-1 State: Protect the health of their citizens by
         1   Special radiological health laws
         2   Nuclear environmental surveillance
         3   Fallout measurements
         4   Radium and x-ray control
         5   Radiation user educational programs
         6   Radiation emergency responses

      7   User control

      8   Complementing the federal aspects of radiation control

      Federal:

      1   Control or delegate to cooperating states source by-product material.

      2   Assist states in terms of research, public information and technical guidance.

      3   Enforce radiation control laws such as PL-90-602, "Radiation Control for Health and Safety Act of 1968."

10-2   To standardize as far as practicable the radiation control regulations in the States.

10-3   U.S. Department of Health, Education and Welfare, Food and Drug Administration: Bureau of Radiological Health.

10-4   1   Repair the unit at no charge to the owner

           2   Replace the unit with one that is in compliance

           3   Refund the cost of the unit to the owner

10-5   The states.

10-6   Under PL-90-602 none. The state has jurisdiction as to the use of the equipment by the owner.

10-7   A visual indication; An audible signal.

10-8   5 min; A signal must indicate the completion of the time and it will remain on until time is reset.

10-9   No; Positive beam-limiting devices are only required on *stationary* general-purpose units.

10-10   Contact your state or local radiation control program director.

Index

Page numbers in **boldface** indicate reference is within an illustration.